# Microbiology and Infectious Diseases *on the move*

# Microbiology and Infectious Diseases *on the move*

Authors: Thomas Locke, Sally Keat, Andrew Walker and Rory Mackinnon
Editorial Advisor: R.C. Read

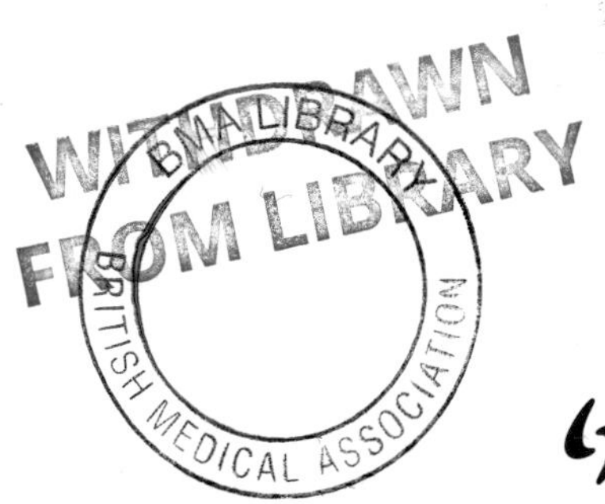


HODDER ARNOLD
AN HACHETTE UK COMPANY

First published in Great Britain in 2012 by
Hodder Arnold, an imprint of Hodder Education, a division of Hachette UK
338 Euston Road, London NW1 3BH

http://www.hodderarnold.com



*British Library Cataloguing in Publication Data*
A catalogue record for this book is available from the British Library

*Library of Congress Cataloging in Publication Data*
A catalog record for this book is available from the Library of Congress

ISBN-13 978-1-444-12012-7

1 2 3 4 5 6 7 8 9 10
Commissioning Editor: Joanna Koster
Project Editor: Stephen Clausard
Production Controller: Francesca Wardell
Cover Design: Amina Dudhia
Indexer: Laurence Errington

Cover image © Sebastian Kaulitzki – Fotolia.com
Typeset in 10/12 pt Adobe Garamond Pro Regular by Datapage
Printed and bound in India by Replika Press

# Contents

# Preface

Ever found medical microbiology and infectious diseases bland and overwhelmingly complicated? Often forget the basics and then struggle with the core texts later on? Or are you simply short of time and have exams looming? If so then this short revision guide will help you. Written by students for students this book presents information in multiple forms including flow charts, colourful diagrams and summary tables. No matter what your learning style, we hope you will find this book appealing and easy to read. We think that this innovative style will help you, the reader, to connect with this often feared topic – hopefully helping you to learn and understand it (maybe even enjoy it!) whilst also helping to bridge the gap to the recommended core texts.

## AUTHORS

**Thomas Locke** BSc MBChB – Foundation Year 1 doctor, Northern General Hospital, Sheffield, UK
**Sally Keat** BMEDSci MBChB – Foundation Year 1 doctor, Northern General Hospital, Sheffield, UK
**Andrew Walker** BMedSci MBChB – Specialist Trainee Year 1 doctor in Medicine, Chesterfield Royal Hospital, Chesterfield, Derbyshire, UK
**Rory Mackinnon** BSc MBChB – Foundation Year 2 doctor, Northern General Hospital, Sheffield, UK

## EDITORIAL ADVISOR

**Professor R.C. Read** – Professor of Infectious Diseases, University of Sheffield, and Honorary Consultant Physician to the Central Sheffield Teaching Hospitals Trust, Royal Hallamshire Hospital, Sheffield, UK

The authors of this title are also the Series Editors for the Medicine on the Move series, with Rory Mackinnon as Editor-in-Chief.

# Acknowledgements

The authors would like to thank the following people for their contribution towards the production of this book:

- Professor Rob Read, University of Sheffield and Central Sheffield Teaching Hospitals, Sheffield, UK.
- Ian Geary, University of Sheffield Medical School, Sheffield, UK.
- Lina Fazlanie and Dr Ian Bickle, Northern General Hospital, Sheffield, UK.
- Centers for Disease Control and Prevention, Atlanta, GA, USA.
- Academic Department of Infection and Immunity, University of Sheffield, UK.

# List of abbreviations

- AIDS: acquired immune deficiency syndrome
- ALT: alanine transaminase
- anti-HBc: anti-hepatitis B core antibody
- anti-HBe: anti-hepatitis B envelope antibody
- anti-HBs: anti-hepatitis B surface antibody
- ARV: anti-retroviral
- AST: aspartate transaminase
- BCG: bacille Calmette–Guérin
- CLO: *Campylobacter*-like organism
- CMV: cytomegalovirus
- COPD: chronic obstructive pulmonary disease
- CRP: c-reactive protein
- CSF: cerebrospinal fluid
- CXR: chest X-ray
- DNA: deoxyribonucleic acid
- dsDNA: double-stranded DNA
- dsRNA: double-stranded RNA
- EBV: Epstein–Barr virus
- ECG: electrocardiogram
- ELISA: enzyme–linked immunosorbent assay
- ESBL: extended spectrum beta-lactamases
- ESR: erythrocyte sedimentation rate
- FBC: full blood count
- FTA-ABS: fluorescent treponemal antibody absorption
- G6PD: glucose-6-phosphate dehydrogenase
- GGT: gamma-glutamyl transferase
- GI: gastrointestinal
- HBeAb: hepatitis B envelope antibody
- HBsAb: hepatitis B suface antibody
- HBeAg: hepatitis B envelope antigen
- HBsAg: hepatitis B surface antigen
- HA: haemagglutinin
- HAART: highly active anti-retroviral therapy
- HAV: hepatitis A virus
- HBV: hepatitis B virus
- HCV: hepatitis C virus
- HDV: hepatitis D virus
- HEV: hepatitis E virus
- HHV: human herpesvirus

- HIV: human immunodeficiency virus
- HSV: herpes simplex virus
- HUS: haemolytic uraemic syndrome
- IFN-$\gamma$: interferon $\gamma$
- Ig: immunoglobulin
- IGRA: interferon-$\gamma$ release assay
- IUGR: intrauterine growth retardation
- IV: intravenous
- IVDU: intravenous drug use
- LFTs: liver function tests
- LP: lumbar puncture
- LRTI: lower respiratory tract infection
- MC&S: microscopy, culture and sensitivity
- MDR-TB: multiple drug-resistant TB
- mRNA: messenger ribonucleic acid
- MRSA: methicillin-resistant *Staphylococcus aureus*
- NA: neuraminidase
- NAD: nicotinamide adenine dinucleotide
- NNRTI: non-nucleoside reverse transcriptase inhibitor
- NRTI: nucleoside reverse transcriptase inhibitor
- NSAID: non-steroidal anti-inflammatory drug
- PBP: penicillin-binding protein
- PCP: *Pneumocystis carinii* pneumonia
- PCR: polymerase chain reaction
- PCV: pneumococcal conjugate vaccine
- PI: protease inhibitors
- PPI: proton pump inhibitor
- RBC: red blood cell
- RNA: ribonucleic acid
- RPR: rapid plasma reagent
- RSV: respiratory syncytial virus
- RT: reverse transcriptase
- RTI: respiratory tract infection
- SLE: systemic lupus erythematosus
- Spp.: species
- ssRNA: single-stranded RNA
- TB: tuberculosis
- TPHA: *T. Pallidum* haemagglutination
- TPPA: *T. Pallidum* particle agglutination
- tRNA: transfer ribonucleic acid
- TSST-1: toxic shock syndrome toxin
- URTI: upper respiratory tract infection
- UTI: urinary tract infection

- VDRL: Venereal Disease Research Laboratory
- VRE: vancomycin-resistant enterococci.
- VZV: varicella zoster virus
- WCC: white cell count
- XDR-TB: extremely drug-resistant TB

# An explanation of the text

The book is divided into three parts: microbiology, infectious diseases and a self-assessment section. We have used bullet points to keep the text concise and brief and supplemented this with a range of diagrams, pictures and MICRO-boxes (explained below).

Where possible we have endeavoured to include treatment options for each condition. Nevertheless, drug sensitivities and clinical practices are constantly under review, so always check your local guidelines for up-to-date information.

**MICRO-facts**

These boxes expand on the text and contain clinically relevant facts and memorable summaries of the essential information.

**MICRO-print**

These boxes contain additional information to the text that may interest certain readers but is not essential for everybody to learn.

**MICRO-case**

These boxes contain clinical cases relevant to the text and include a number of summary bullet points to highlight the key learning objectives.

**MICRO-reference**

These boxes contain references to important clinical research and national guidance.

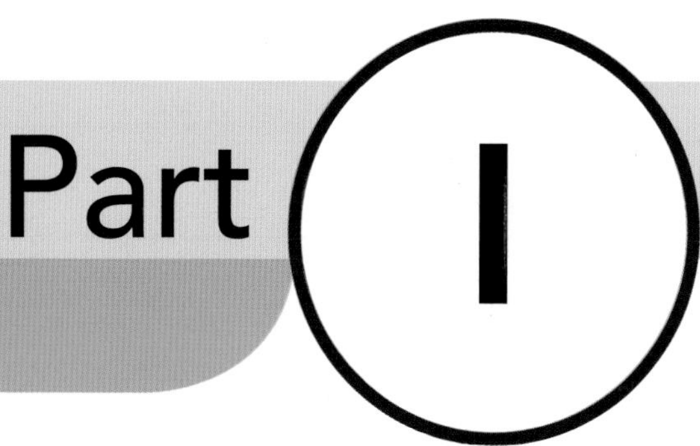


# Microbiology

# 1 Bacteria

## 1.1 BACTERIAL STRUCTURE

### MICRO-facts

Bacteria are prokaryotes – cells with deoxyribonucleic acid (DNA) free within the cytoplasm.

Eukaryotes are cells with a nucleus containing their DNA, e.g. fungi, amoebae.

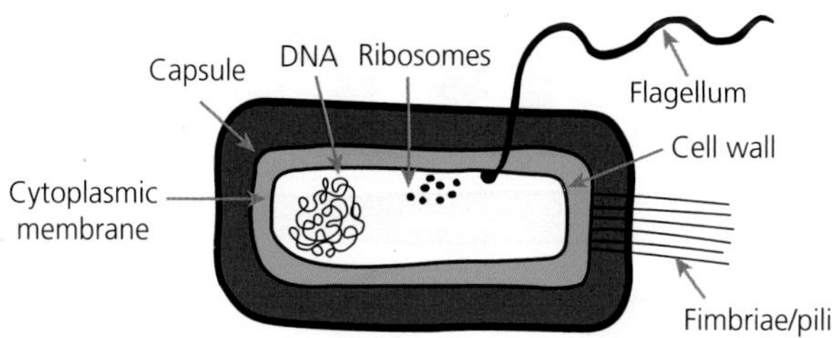


Fig. 1.1 Generic bacterial structure.

### CAPSULE

- Outermost layer of bacteria.
- Provides protection by preventing phagocytosis.
- Not found on all bacteria.

### CELL WALL

- Strong outer cover that maintains bacterial shape and protects against osmotic pressure.
- Variations in cell wall structure account for Gram-positive and Gram-negative staining (a method used to classify and identify bacteria):
  - **Gram positive**: thick peptidoglycan layer (repeating sugar subunits cross-linked by peptide chains) in the cell wall.

- **Gram negative**: thin peptidoglycan layer and an additional outer membrane containing lipopolysaccharides (also called endotoxin).

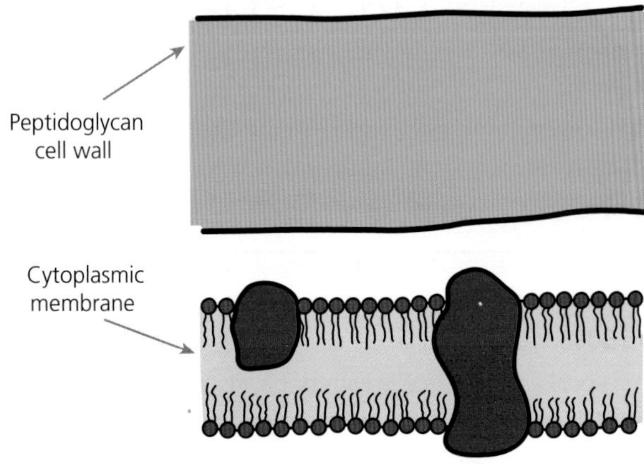


Fig. 1.2 Gram-positive cell wall and cytoplasmic membrane.

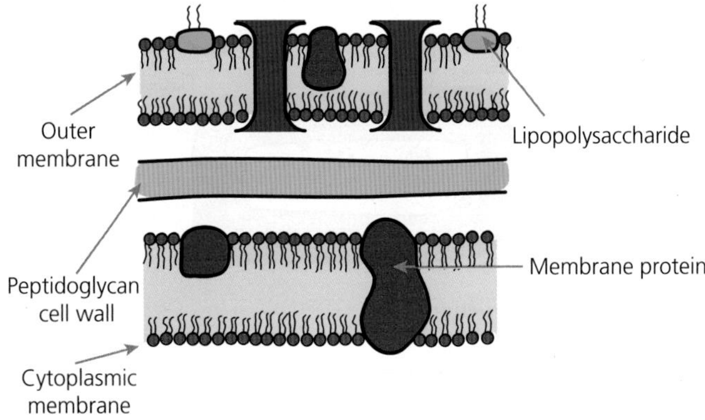


Fig. 1.3 Gram-negative cell wall and cytoplasmic membrane.

## CYTOPLASMIC MEMBRANE

- Phospholipid bilayer with embedded proteins.
- Surrounds the cytoplasm.
- A semipermeable membrane that regulates the movement of substances in and out of the bacteria.

## FLAGELLA

- Spiral-shaped filaments that allow movement.

- Formed by multiple subunits of flagellin (a protein).

### FIMBRIAE/PILI

- Shorter than flagella.
- Arise from the cytoplasmic membrane.
- Formed by multiple subunits of pilin (a protein).
- Allow the bacteria to adhere to cell surfaces and exchange plasmids (containing genetic material) with other bacteria.

### DEOXYRIBONUCLEIC ACID

- Single circular strand of double-stranded deoxyribonucleic acid (DNA).
- No nuclear membrane, free within cytoplasm.

### RIBOSOMES

- Site of protein synthesis within the cytoplasm.

### PLASMIDS

- Double-stranded circular DNA molecules found in some bacteria.
- Genes within the plasmid may confer an advantage for the bacteria such as antibiotic resistance or exotoxins.
- Can be transferred between bacteria.

## 1.2 OXYGEN REQUIREMENTS

Bacteria have a range of oxygen requirements.

### AEROBES

- **Obligate aerobes**: require oxygen to grow (e.g. *Mycobacterium tuberculosis*).
- **Microaerophilic**: optimal growth in low oxygen concentrations (e.g. *Campylobacter* spp. at 5% $O_2$).

### ANAEROBES

- **Obligate anaerobes**: require an oxygen-free environment to grow (e.g. *Clostridium* spp.).
- **Facultative anaerobes**: can grow in aerobic or anaerobic conditions (e.g. *Bacillus* spp.).

## 1.3 BACTERIAL CLASSIFICATION AND IDENTIFICATION

Bacteria can be classified and identified by **shape, staining, biochemical tests, sensitivity tests, culture techniques**, **serological tests** and **nucleic acid techniques.**

## BACTERIAL SHAPES

- Cocci (spheres).
- Bacilli (rods).
- Vibrio (curved rod).
- Spirochaete (spiral rod).

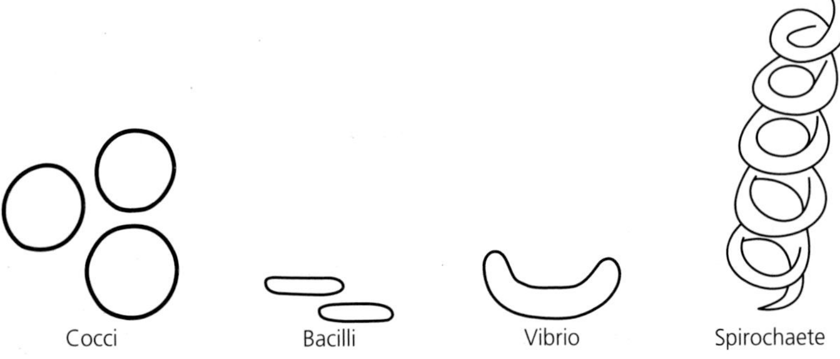


Fig. 1.4 Bacterial shapes.

## BACTERIAL STAINING

> **MICRO-facts**
>
> Gram-**p**ositive bacteria stain **purple**.

### Gram staining

- Gram staining classifies bacteria into two groups:
  - **Gram positive**: **purple** – thick peptidoglycan layer in cell wall retains methyl violet.
  - **Gram negative**: **red** – alcohol dissolves cell wall lipids and methyl violet stain is lost, basic fuchsin then counterstains Gram-negative bacteria red.
- Fungi and pus cells (neutrophils) will also be visible after a Gram stain.
- Technique:
  - heat fix sample to the slide;
  - add methyl violet (blue/purple);
  - add iodine; this will fix the methyl violet to Gram-positive samples;
  - add alcohol to decolour Gram-negative samples;
  - counterstain with basic fuchsin (red).

### Ziehl–Neelsen staining

- Identifies acid-fast bacteria:
  - ***Mycobacteria* spp. (acid fast)**: **pink/red**;
  - **non-acid fast** bacteria: **blue**.
- Gram staining cannot be used as cell wall contains mycolic acids (lipids), making the bacteria impermeable to the dyes.

> **MICRO-facts**
>
> *Mycobacteria* spp. are acid fast: they stain pink/red with Ziehl–Neelsen staining.

### Auramine–rhodamine stain

- Identifies acid-fast bacteria.
- Used more frequently than Ziehl–Neelsen staining.
- The dye binds with *Mycobacteria* spp. and turns them bright yellow when viewed with fluorescence microscopy.

## BIOCHEMICAL TESTS

### Catalase test

- Differentiates between:
  - **staphylococci**: catalase **positive**;
  - **streptococci** and **enterococci**: catalase **negative**.
- Catalase is an enzyme that catalyses the following reaction:

$$2H_2O_2 \rightarrow 2H_2O + O_2$$

$$\text{Hydrogen peroxide} \rightarrow \text{Water} + \text{Oxygen}$$

- *Staphylococcus* spp. use catalase to protect against hydrogen peroxide ($H_2O_2$) by converting it into water and oxygen; therefore:

$$H_2O_2 + \text{Staphylococci} \rightarrow \text{Gas bubbles}$$

$$H_2O_2 + \text{Streptococci/enterococci} \rightarrow \text{No reaction}$$

> **MICRO-facts**
>
> **Catalase** test:
>
> **Bubbles** (positive) = **staphylococci**.
>
> **No bubbles** (negative) = **streptococci/enterococci** spp.

Microbiology

### Coagulase test

- Differentiates between:
  - ***Staphylococcus aureus***: coagulase **positive**.
  - Other ***Staphylococcus*** spp.: coagulase **negative**.
- Coagulase is an enzyme that causes plasma to clot by converting fibrinogen into fibrin, preventing phagocytosis.

*Staphylococcus aureus* + Plasma → Clot

Other *Staphylococcus* spp. + Plasma → No clot

> **MICRO-facts**
>
> **Coagulase** test:
>
> **Clot** (positive) = ***Staphylococcus aureus***.
>
> **No clot** (negative) = Other ***Staphylococcus*** spp.

### Oxidase test

- Identifies bacteria that are oxidase positive, i.e. they produce cytochrome oxidase:
  - ***Pseudomonas*** spp.;
  - ***Neisseria*** spp.;
  - ***Vibrio*** spp.
- Oxidase-positive bacteria produce cytochrome oxidase, which enables them to oxidase certain amine-containing reagents.

*Pseudomonas* spp. or *Neisseria* spp. or *Vibrio* spp. + Reagent
→ Black-ish/Purple colour

Oxidase-negative bacteria + Reagent → No colour change

### Urease tests

- Differentiate between:
  - ***Helicobacter pylori***: urease positive.
  - ***Campylobacter*** spp.: urease negative.
- *H. pylori* produces urease, an enzyme that enables the organism to split urea and form ammonia.
- This property of *H. pylori* forms the basis of the following diagnostic biochemical tests:
  - **$^{13}$C-Urea breath test**: ingested $^{13}$C-urea is converted to $^{13}CO_2$, which is detected in the patient's breath by a mass spectrometer. Ammonia is also produced.

- **Rapid urease test**: a gastric biopsy is obtained during endoscopy and added to a solution of urea. If *H. pylori* is present, ammonia is produced and a pH indicator detects this alkaline environment.

## SENSITIVITY TESTS

### Optochin test

- Differentiates between:
    - ***Streptococcus pneumoniae***: cell **lysis**.
    - **Other α-haemolytic streptococci** (*viridans*): no **lysis**.
- Optochin is a chemical that causes lysis of *S. pneumoniae*.

*Streptococcus pneumoniae* + Optochin
→ Lysis (zone of inhibition)

Other α-haemolytic streptococci (*viridans*) + Optochin
→ No lysis

> **MICRO-facts**
>
> Optochin inhibits the growth of *Streptococcus pneumoniae*. It does not affect other α-haemolytic streptococci.

### Metronidazole

- Identifies sensitive anaerobes by inhibiting their growth on culture medium.

### Antibiotic sensitivity

- Discs impregnated with antibiotics placed on culture samples can reveal sensitivity and resistance.
- Used to guide clinical management, especially when antibiotic-resistant strains are prevalent.

## CULTURE TECHNIQUES

### MacConkey agar

- Isolates and identifies enteric bacteria.
- Contains bile salts, lactose and pH indicator:
    - **Bile salts**: only permit the growth of enteric bacteria (isolation).
    - **Lactose and pH indicator**: fermentation of lactose produces an acidic environment that causes the pH indicator to become red/pink (identification):
        - **Red/pink colony**: ***Escherichia coli*** and **Klebsiella** spp.
        - **Clear colony** (no fermentation): ***Salmonella*** spp., ***Shigella*** spp., ***Proteus*** spp. and ***Pseudomonas*** spp.

> **MICRO-facts**
>
> MacConkey agar:
>
> **Red/pink** = *Escherichia coli* or *Klebsiella* spp.
>
> Clear = *Salmonella* spp., *Shigella* spp., *Proteus* spp. or *Pseudomonas* spp.

### Blood agar

- Differentiates between:
  - **α-haemolytic** *Streptococcus* spp.;
  - **β-haemolytic** *Streptococcus* spp.;
  - **γ-haemolytic** *Streptococcus* spp.
- Contains mammalian blood.
- α,β and γ strains have different effects on the blood:
  - **α-Haemolytic**: **partial** erythrocyte and haemoglobin breakdown releases a **green** pigment.
  - **β-Haemolytic**: **complete** erythrocyte lysis results in **clear** zones.
  - **γ-Haemolytic**: no change.

> **MICRO-facts**
>
> Blood agar:
>
> **Green** = α-haemolytic *Streptococcus* spp.
>
> Clear = β-haemolytic *Streptococcus* spp.
>
> No change = γ-haemolytic *Streptococcus* spp.

### Lowenstein–Jensen medium

- Medium used to culture *Mycobacterium* spp.
- Contains egg yolk and glycerol to facilitate *Mycobacterium* spp. growth and malachite green to minimize the growth of other bacteria.
- The culture process can take up to 12 weeks as *Mycobacterium* spp. replicate slowly.

### Chocolate agar with factor V and X discs

- *Haemophilus influenzae* will only grow on agar containing factor V (nicotinamide adenine dinucleotide or NAD) and factor X (haematin).

### Charcoal blood agar

- Medium used to culture *Bordetella pertussis.*
- Contains charcoal and mammalian blood.

### Buffered charcoal yeast extract agar

- Medium used to culture *Legionella* spp.
- Contains high concentrations of iron and cysteine.

### Chocolate agar plates

- Medium used to culture *H. pylori.*
- Similar to blood agar except the red blood cells have been lysed by heating.
- This process results in the characteristic chocolate colour.

### Blood tellurite agar

- Medium used to culture *Corynebacterium diphtheriae.*
- Contains potassium tellurite salt and mammalian blood.
- *C. diphtheriae* reduce the potassium tellurite salt to tellurium, which has a grey–black colour.

## SEROLOGICAL TESTS

### Lancefield grouping

- Differentiates between β-haemolytic *Streptococcus* spp. by detecting surface antigens.
- Three medically important groups:
  - **A**: *Streptococcus pyogenes.*
  - **B**: *Streptococcus agalactiae.*
  - **D**: now reclassified as *Enterococcus* genus.

### Enzyme-linked immunosorbent assay

- Used to detect the presence of antigen or antibody in a patient's sample.
- **Antigen**:
  - Complementary antibodies to the suspected antigen are attached to slides.
  - The patient's sample (e.g. respiratory secretions) is added to the slides and, if the viral antigen is present, an antibody–antigen complex will form.
  - This can be demonstrated by adding a second antibody with an attached enzyme.
  - When enzyme substrate is added, the subsequent enzyme activity can be detected (e.g. the colour of the solution may change).
- **Antibody**:
  - Microtitration trays with multiple wells are precoated with the suspected microbial antigen.
  - The patient's sample is added and, if the antibodies are present, an antigen–antibody complex will form.

   - Antibody (with attached enzyme) to human immunoglobulin is then added and binds with the antigen–antibody complex.
   - Enzyme substrate can then be added as described above.
- See Fig. 1.5.

### Immunofluorescence

- Uses a similar theory to enzyme-linked immunosorbent assay (ELISA) but a fluorescent dye is attached to the antibody or antigen molecules instead of an enzyme.
- If the corresponding antigen/antibody is present in the sample then an antigen–antibody complex will form and the dye will be visible when using a fluorescent microscope.

### Agglutination

- When an antigen is added to a sample containing antibodies, multiple bonds are formed that result in a mesh.
- Macroscopically, clumping of the sample can be seen.
- This method is used to determine ABO blood groups or diagnose syphilis (non-specific test).

### Protein A

- Differentiates between:
   - ***S. aureus***: protein A present.
   - **Other *Staphylococcus*** spp.: protein A negative.
- Protein A forms part of the cell wall of *S. aureus* and protects the bacterium against opsonization and phagocytosis by inactivating the complement binding site.
- ELISA testing can detect protein A.

## NUCLEIC ACID TECHNIQUES

### Polymerase chain reaction

- Polymerase chain reaction (PCR) can be used to detect a broad range of organisms including bacteria, viruses and fungi.
- The process of PCR results in a significant increase in the amount of microbial DNA or ribonucleic acid obtained from a patient sample.
- This genetic material can then be examined for sections that are specific to a certain organism.
- PCR is particularly helpful for detecting slow-growing organisms or those that are difficult to culture.

# 1.4 TOXINS

Bacteria produce two types of toxin: **exotoxin** and **endotoxin**. See Table 1.1.

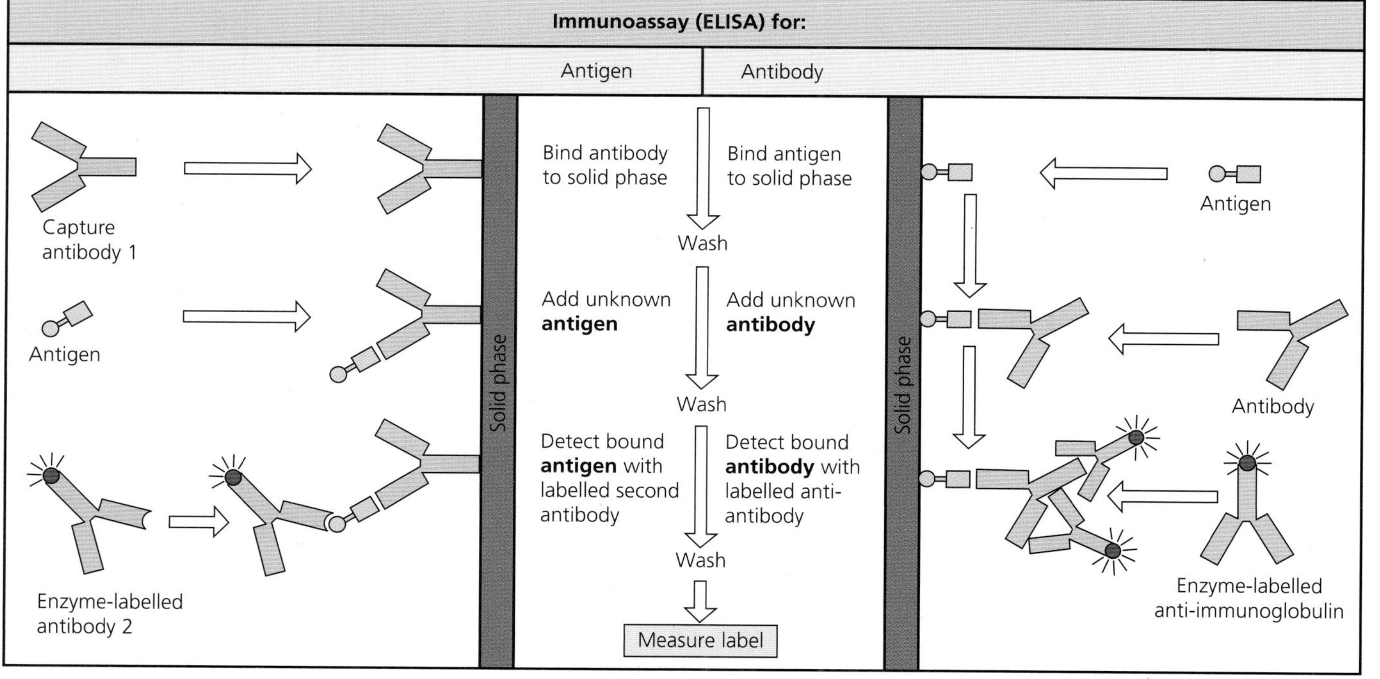


Fig. 1.5 Enzyme-linked immunosorbent assay testing for antigens and antibodies. (Reprinted with permission from Goering R, Dockrell H, Zuckerman M *et al. Mim's Medical Microbiology*, 4th edn. Copyright Elsevier 2007.)

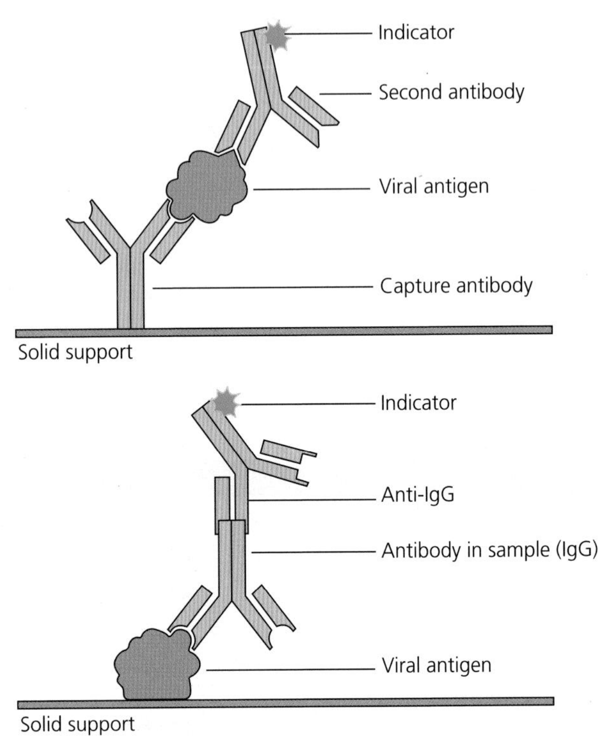


Fig. 1.5 *(Continued)*

Table 1.1 Comparison of bacterial exotoxin and endotoxin

| CHARACTERISTIC | EXOTOXIN | ENDOTOXIN |
|---|---|---|
| Production | Actively secreted by bacteria | Cell wall component, released when the bacterium is damaged |
| Composition | Protein | Lipopolysaccharide |
| Gram positive/negative | Gram positive and negative | Gram negative |
| Mode of action | Specific action | Non-specific, e.g. sepsis |
| Examples | *Clostridium tetani* (tetanospasmin) *Bordetella pertussis* (pertussis toxin) | All Gram-negative bacteria have the potential to produce endotoxin |

## 1.5 GRAM-POSITIVE BACTERIA IDENTIFICATION FLOWCHART (FIG. 1.6)

## 1.6 GRAM-POSITIVE BACTERIA

There are six key groups of Gram-positive (purple/blue staining) bacteria:

1. *Streptococcus* spp.;
2. *Staphylococcus* spp.;
3. *Corynebacterium* spp.;
4. *Listeria* spp.;
5. *Bacillus* spp.;
6. *Clostridium* spp.

**MICRO-facts**

The **six Gram-positive** bacteria can be remembered with this **mnemonic**:

| | |
|---|---|
| **S**exy | ***S**treptococcus* spp. |
| **S**tudents | ***S**taphylococcus* spp. |
| **C**an | ***C**orynebacterium* spp. |
| **L**ook | ***L**isteria* spp. |
| **B**ad | ***B**acillus* spp. |
| **C**ome the morning | ***C**lostridium* spp. |

### *STREPTOCOCCUS* SPP.

#### Characteristics

- **Shape**: chains except for *S. pneumoniae* (diplococci, pairs of cocci).
- **Staining**: Gram-positive.
- **Biochemical tests**:
  - **Catalase test**: catalase negative.
- **Sensitivity tests**:
  - Optochin test:
    - **Optochin positive**: *S. pneumoniae.*
    - **Optochin negative**: other α-haemolytic *Streptococcus* spp. (*viridans* group).
- **Culture techniques**:
  - **Blood agar**:
    - **Green** (α-haemolytic *Streptococcus* spp.):
      - *S. pneumoniae.*
      - *viridans* group (broad range of bacteria): *Streptococcus oralis*; *Streptococcus sanguis*; *Streptococcus mutans*; *Streptococcus mitis.*

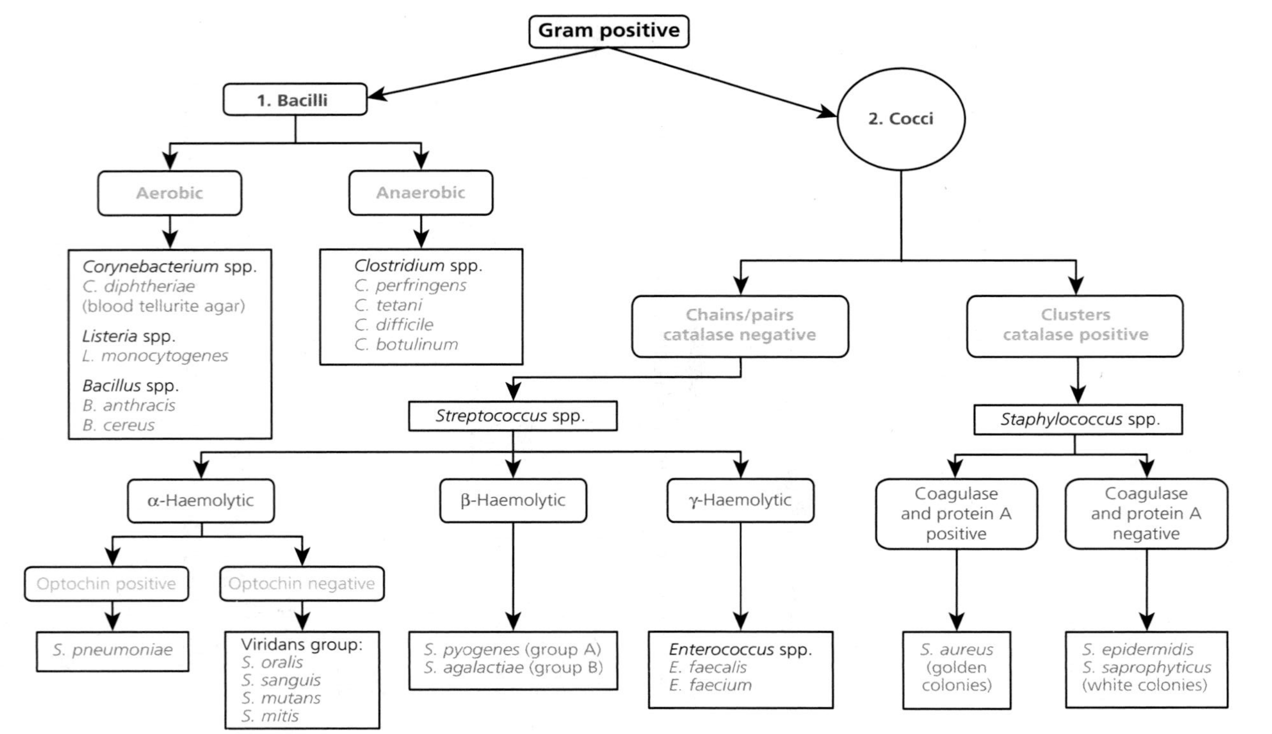


Fig. 1.6 Gram-positive bacteria identification flowchart.

- **Clear zone** (β-haemolytic *Streptococcus* spp.):
  - *S. pyogenes* (group A);
  - *S. agalactiae* (group B).
- **No change** (γ-haemolytic *Streptococcus* spp.):
  - *Enterococcus faecalis*;
  - *Enterococcus faecium*.

- **Serological tests**:
  - **Lancefield grouping**:
    - **A**: *S. pyogenes*.
    - **B**: *S. agalactiae*.
    - **D**: many reclassified to *Enterococcus* genus (two most important species are *E. faecalis* and *E. faecium)*.
- **Oxygen requirement**: aerobic.

## Key examples

### Streptococcus pneumoniae *(pneumococcus) (α-haemolytic)*

- **Location**: commensal of upper respiratory tract in 10–30%.
- **Transmission**: respiratory droplet spread.
- **Diseases**:
  - **Respiratory**: pneumonia (community acquired), chronic obstructive pulmonary disease (COPD) exacerbation and sinusitis (see Chapter 7, Respiratory infections).
  - **Neurological**: meningitis (see Chapter 12, Nervous system infections).
  - **Ophthalmic**: conjunctivitis.
  - **Blood**: septicaemia.
  - **ENT**: otitis media.
  - **Post-splenectomy**: increased risk of pneumococcal infection secondary to reduced immunoglobulin M (IgM) antibody production.
- **Anti-microbial**:
  - **Resistance**: penicillins, macrolides and doxycycline.
  - **Respiratory**:
    - **Pneumonia**: amoxicillin, benzylpenicillin (no previous chest pathology) or erythromycin (penicillin allergy).
    - **COPD exacerbation**: amoxicillin or a tetracycline or erythromycin.
    - **Sinusitis**: amoxicillin, doxycycline or erythromycin (only treat symptoms lasting more than 7 days or those at high risk of complications).
  - **Neurological**:
    - **Meningitis**: third-generation cephalosporin or a penicillin (if known to be sensitive).
  - **Ophthalmic**:
    - **Conjunctivitis**: chloramphenicol or gentamicin.

- **Blood**:
  - **Sepsis**: third-generation cephalosporin or a penicillin (if known to be sensitive).
- **ENT**:
  - **Otitis media**: amoxicillin or erythromycin (penicillin allergy) (many cases resolve without treatment; use antibiotics if no improvement after 72 hours, systemic features, high risk of complications or mastoiditis present).
- **Splenectomy**: phenoxymethylpenicillin (penicillin V) prophylaxis.
- **Immunization**:
  - **UK schedule**: 2, 3 and 13 months of age.
  - Splenectomy.
  - Over 65 years old (recommended).

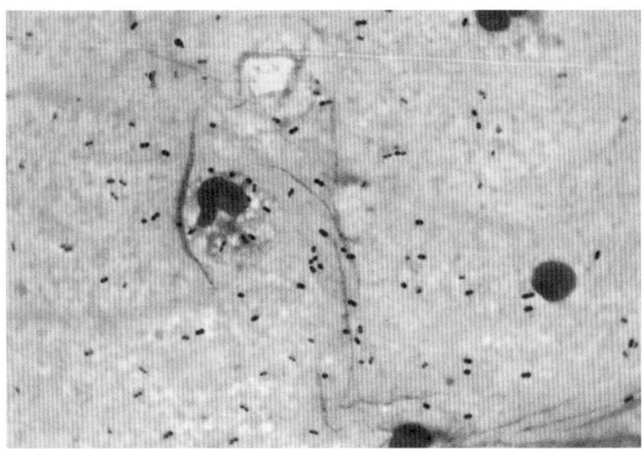

Fig. 1.7 *Streptococcus pneumoniae* stained with Gram stain. Courtesy of the Academic Department of Infection & Immunity, University of Sheffield, UK.

Viridans streptococci *(α-haemolytic)*

- **Location**: upper respiratory tract, gastrointestinal tract and oral cavity commensal.
- **Transmission**: enter the bloodstream during dental procedures.
- **Diseases**:
  - **Cardiovascular**: infective endocarditis (particularly after dental manipulation) (see Chapter 9, Cardiovascular infections).
  - **Dental**: dental caries (especially *S. mutans*).
- **Anti-microbial**:
  - **Cardiovascular**:
    - **Infective endocarditis**: benzylpenicillin or vancomycin (penicillin allergy) and gentamicin.

### Streptococcus pyogenes *(group A $\beta$-haemolytic)*

- **Location**: upper respiratory tract commensals in 5% of adults and 10% of children.
- **Transmission**: respiratory droplet spread and skin contact.
- **Diseases**:
  - **Skin**: cellulitis, necrotizing fasciitis, impetigo, erysipelas and wound infections (see Chapter 13, Skin infections).
  - **ENT**: otitis media, pharyngitis ('strep throat') and tonsillitis.
  - **Toxins**: toxic shock syndrome and scarlet fever.
  - **Blood**: septicaemia.
  - **Post-infective**: rheumatic fever, post-streptococcal glomerulonephritis; associated with guttate psoriasis.
- **Anti-microbial**:
  - **Resistance**: increasing resistance to erythromycin.
  - **Skin**: benzylpenicillin or phenoxymethylpenicillin.
  - **ENT**: see Chapter 7, Respiratory infections.
    - **Otitis media**: amoxicillin or erythromycin (if penicillin allergic) (many cases resolve without treatment; use antibiotics if no improvement after 72 hours, systemic features, high risk of complications or mastoiditis present).
    - **Pharyngitis**: phenoxymethylpenicillin or erythromycin (if penicillin allergic).
    - **Tonsillitis**: phenoxymethylpenicillin or erythromycin (if penicillin allergic).
  - **Toxin mediated**:
    - **Toxic shock syndrome**: benzylpenicillin or clindamycin (see Chapter 11, Genitourinary infections).
    - **Scarlet fever**: benzylpenicillin or phenoxymethylpenicillin or erythromycin (if penicillin allergic).
  - **Post-infective**:
    - **Rheumatic fever**: benzylpenicillin or erythromycin (if penicillin allergic) (see Chapter 9, Cardiovascular infections).

### Streptococcus agalactiae *(group B $\beta$-haemolytic)*

- **Location**: faecal (30–40% of population) and female genital tract commensal (10–30% of population).
- **Transmission**: during labour.
- **Diseases**:
  - **Neurological**: meningitis (especially neonates).
  - **Blood**: septicaemia.
  - **Cardiovascular**: infective endocarditis.
  - **Obstetric**: septic abortion and postpartum sepsis.

- **Anti-microbial**:
  - **Neurological**: see Chapter 12, Nervous system infections.
    - **Meningitis**: benzylpenicillin (community) or cefotaxime.
  - **Blood**:
    - **Septicaemia**: benzylpenicillin or amoxicillin.
  - **Cardiovascular**: see Chapter 9, Cardiovascular infections.
    - **Infective endocarditis**: benzylpenicillin or vancomycin (penicillin allergy) and gentamicin.

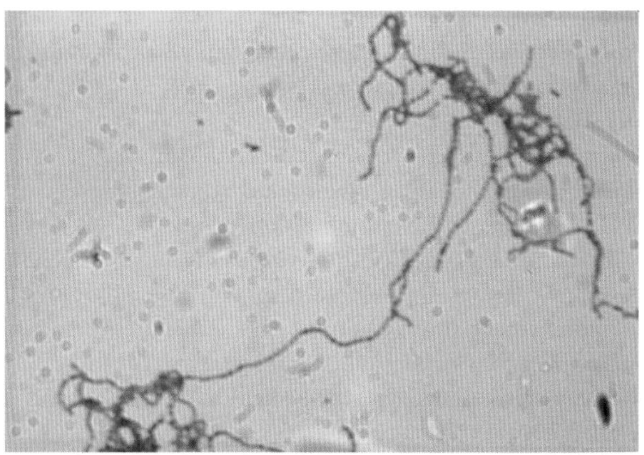

Fig. 1.8 Streptococci in characteristic chains, stained with Gram stain. Courtesy of the Academic Department of Infection & Immunity, University of Sheffield, UK.

### Enterococcus *spp. (group D γ-haemolytic)*

- Formerly group D *Streptococcus*, now separate genus.
- **Location**: gastrointestinal tract commensal.
- **Diseases**:
  - **Urinary tract**: urinary tract infection (UTI) (see Chapter 11, Genitourinary infections).
  - **Cardiovascular**: infective endocarditis (see Chapter 9, Cardiovascular infections).
  - **Skin**: wound infections and intravenous (IV) line infection (see Chapter 13, Skin infections).
- **Anti-microbial**:
  - **Resistance**: increasing resistance to gentamicin and vancomycin (vancomycin-resistant enterococci (VRE)).
  - **Urinary tract**:
    - **UTI**: amoxicillin or nitrofurantoin.

- **Cardiovascular**:
  - **Infective endocarditis**: amoxicillin or vancomycin (penicillin allergy) and gentamicin.
- **Skin**:
  - **Wound and IV line infection**: amoxicillin.

> **MICRO-facts**
>
> Shape:
>
> *Staphylococcus* spp. = cocci clumps.
>
> *Streptococcus* spp. = cocci chains (except *S. pneumoniae* = diplococci).

## *STAPHYLOCOCCUS* SPP.

### Characteristics

- **Shape**: cocci in clumps (like grapes).
- **Characteristic morphology**:
  - **Golden yellow colonies**: *S. aureus* (an aureus was a gold coin used in ancient Rome).
  - **White colonies**: *Staphylococcus epidermidis* and *Staphylococcus saprophyticus*.
- **Staining**: Gram-positive.
- **Biochemical tests**:
  - **Catalase test**: catalase positive.
  - **Coagulase test**:
    - **Coagulase positive**: *S. aureus*.
    - **Coagulase negative**:
      - *S. epidermidis*;
      - *S. saprophyticus*.
- **Serological tests**:
  - **Protein A**:
    - **Positive**: *S. aureus*.
    - **Negative**: coagulase-negative staphylococci.
- **Oxygen requirement**: aerobic.

> **MICRO-facts**
>
> **MRSA** is **m**ethicillin (prototype flucloxacillin)-**r**esistant ***S**taphylococcus **a**ureus*.

## Key examples

### Staphylococcus aureus

- **Location**:
  - anterior nares in 20–30% of the general population;
  - skin, in particular axilla and perineum;
  - gastrointestinal tract;
  - vagina.
- **Transmission**: skin contact.
- **Diseases**:
  - **Skin**: impetigo, paronychia, abscesses, cellulitis, wound/IV line infection (see Chapter 13, Skin infections).
  - **Bones and joints**: osteomyelitis and septic arthritis (see Chapter 14, Bone and joint infections).
  - **Respiratory**: pneumonia (especially post-influenza or measles infection) (see Chapter 7, Respiratory infections).
  - **Blood**: septicaemia.
  - **Ophthalmic**: conjunctivitis.
  - **Cardiovascular**: infective endocarditis (frequently among intravenous drug users) (see Chapter 9, Cardiovascular infections).
  - **Toxin mediated**: toxic shock syndrome, scalded skin syndrome and gastroenteritis (see Chapters 8, Gastrointestinal infections; 11, Genitourinary infections; 13, Skin infections).
- **Anti-microbial**:
  - **Sensitivities**: flucloxacillin.
  - **Resistance**: methicillin/flucloxacillin (MRSA).
  - **Skin**:
    - **Impetigo**: flucloxacillin (oral).
    - **Cellulitis**: flucloxacillin.
  - **Bones and joints**:
    - **Osteomyelitis and septic arthritis**: flucloxacillin or clindamycin (penicillin allergy) or vancomycin (MRSA).
  - **Respiratory**:
    - **Pneumonia**: amoxicillin or benzylpenicillin (previously healthy chest) or **erythromycin** (penicillin allergy) and flucloxacillin.
  - **Blood**:
    - **Septicaemia**: flucloxacillin or vancomycin (MRSA).
  - **Ophthalmic**:
    - **Conjunctivitis**: chloramphenicol or gentamicin eye drops.
  - **Cardiovascular**:
    - **Infective endocarditis**: flucloxacillin or vancomycin and rifampicin (penicillin allergy or MRSA).

**MICRO-print**

***STAPHYLOCOCCUS AUREUS***

***S. aureus*** bacteria produce multiple pathogenic **toxins**:
**Toxic shock syndrome toxin:** toxic shock syndrome.
**Exfoliatin:** scalded skin syndrome.
**Enterotoxin:** gastroenteritis.
**Panton–Valentine leucocidin:** pyogenic skin infections or pneumonia (destroys white blood cells).

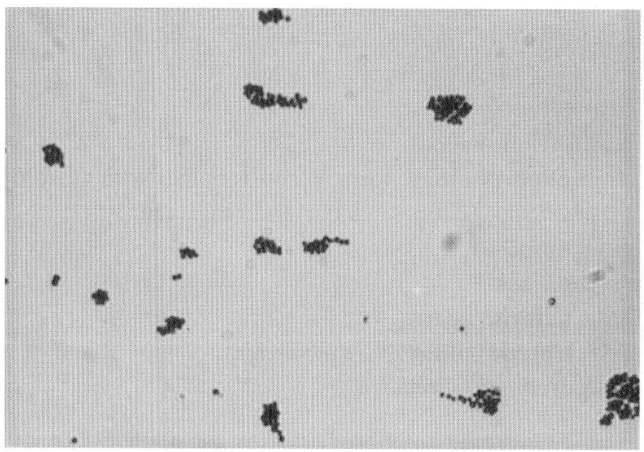

Fig. 1.9 *Staphylococcus aureus* stained with Gram stain. Courtesy of the Academic Department of Infection & Immunity, University of Sheffield, UK.

### Staphylococcus epidermidis

- **Location**: skin and mucous membranes.
- **Transmission**: infection usually with own flora or skin contact.
- **Diseases**:
    - Mostly harmless commensal that causes disease under special circumstances, especially post-surgery or in patients with prostheses.
    - **Prostheses**: prostheses (e.g. prosthetic heart valves and joints) and IV line infection.
    - **Cardiovascular**: infective endocarditis (see Chapter 9, Cardiovascular infections).
- **Anti-microbial**:
    - **Cardiovascular**:
        - **Infective endocarditis**: flucloxacillin or vancomycin and rifampicin (penicillin allergy or MRSA).

### Staphylococcus saprophyticus

- **Location**: peri-genitourinary tract skin.
- **Transmission**: infection usually with own flora.
- **Diseases**:
  - **Urinary tract**: UTI (the commonest cause of honeymoon cystitis, so named because of its high prevalence among sexually active young women) (see Chapter 11, Genitourinary infections).
- **Anti-microbial**:
  - **Urinary tract**:
    - **UTI**: trimethoprim or nitrofurantoin or amoxicillin or oral cephalosporin.

## *CORYNEBACTERIUM* SPP.

### Characteristics

- **Shape**: bacilli (club shaped).
- **Characteristic morphology**: form V and L shapes with adjacent *Corynebacterium* spp. (Chinese character arrangement).
- **Staining**: Gram-positive.
- **Culture techniques**:
  - **Blood tellurite agar**:
    - **Grey/black colony**: *C. diphtheriae.*
- **Oxygen requirement**: aerobic.

### Key example

> **MICRO-facts**
>
> Diphtheria toxin causes epithelial cell destruction and myocardial/neural cell damage.

### Corynebacterium diphtheriae

- **Location**: nasopharynx.
- **Transmission**: respiratory droplet spread.
- **Diseases**: diphtheria (sore throat with grey-white pseudomembrane covering the fauces and lymphadenopathy with bull neck appearance).
- **Anti-microbial**:
  - **Diphtheria**: benzylpenicillin or erythromycin and diphtheria anti-toxin (in hospital).
  - **Immunization (UK schedule)**: 2, 3 and 4 months, 3 years and 4 months, and 13–18 years old.

## *LISTERIA* SPP.

### Characteristics

- **Shape**: bacilli.
- **Characteristic morphology**: forms V and L shape arrangements with adjacent *Listeria* spp.
- **Staining**: Gram-positive.
- **Oxygen requirement**: facultative anaerobe.

### Key example

#### Listeria monocytogenes

- **Location**:
  - gastrointestinal tract;
  - vagina;
  - domestic animal faeces;
  - food (e.g. soft cheese, unpasteurized milk).
- **Transmission**: contact with animals, ingestion, *in utero* or perinatally.
- **Diseases**:
  - **Obstetric**: miscarriage, stillbirth or neonatal death (see Chapter 15, Congenital, neonatal and childhood infections).
  - **Neurological**: meningitis or encephalitis (especially neonates or immunocompromised) (see Chapter 12, Nervous system infections).
  - **Respiratory**: pneumonia.
  - **Blood**: septicaemia.
- **Anti-microbial**:
  - **Listeriosis**: amoxicillin or erythromycin (if penicillin allergic).
  - **Neurological**:
    - **Meningitis and encephalitis**: amoxicillin and gentamicin.

## *BACILLUS* SPP.

### Characteristics

- **Shape**: bacilli.
- **Characteristic morphology**: spore forming.
- **Staining**: Gram-positive.
- **Oxygen requirement**: facultatively anaerobic.

### Key examples

#### Bacillus anthracis

- **Location**:
  - infected herbivore carcasses;
  - soil.

- **Transmission**: skin exposure to spores, spore inhalation or ingestion.
- **Diseases**:
  - **Anthrax**:
    - **Cutaneous**: painless lesions with central necrosis (black eschar), local lymphadenopathy and systemic malaise.
    - **Pulmonary**: flu-like illness, shortness of breath and respiratory failure.
    - **Gastrointestinal**: abdominal pain, vomiting and diarrhoea (watery or bloody).
- **Anti-microbial**:
  - **Cutaneous anthrax**: ciprofloxacin or doxycycline.
  - **Pulmonary and gastrointestinal anthrax**: ciprofloxacin or doxycycline and one or two from amoxicillin, benzylpenicillin, chloramphenicol, clarithromycin, clindamycin, imipenem, rifampicin or vancomycin.

### Bacillus cereus

- **Location**: foods (especially rice).
- **Transmission**: spores can survive cooking temperatures and replicate when kept warm (such as improperly refrigerated food). Ingested spores release toxin that causes gastrointestinal disease.
- **Diseases**:
  - **Gastrointestinal**: gastroenteritis (see Chapter 8, Gastrointestinal infections).
- **Anti-microbial**: self-limiting disease.

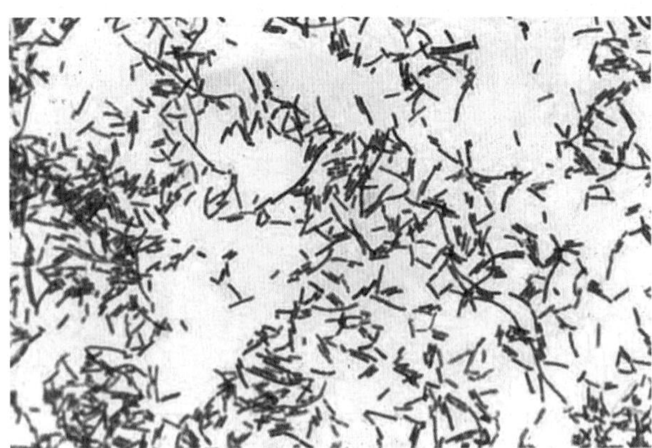

Fig. 1.10 *Bacillus cereus* stained with Gram stain. Courtesy of the Academic Department of Infection & Immunity, University of Sheffield, UK.

## *CLOSTRIDIUM* SPP.

### Characteristics

- **Shape**: bacilli.
- **Characteristic morphology**:
  - Spore forming.
  - **Brick shaped**: *Clostridium perfringens.*
  - **Terminal spores**: *Clostridium tetani* (resembles tennis racket or drumstick).
- **Staining**: Gram-positive.
- **Biochemical tests**:
  - **Toxin**: *Clostridium difficile* toxins can be detected in stool samples.
- **Oxygen requirement**: anaerobic.

### Key examples

#### Clostridium perfringens

- **Location**:
  - human and animal gastrointestinal tracts;
  - soil.
- **Transmission**:
  - wound contamination with soil or gastrointestinal contents;
  - ingestion of contaminated food (endotoxin released after ingestion).
- **Diseases**:
  - **Skin**: gas gangrene (see Chapter 13, Skin infections).
  - **Gastrointestinal**: gastroenteritis (see Chapter 8, Gastrointestinal infections).
- **Anti-microbial**:
  - **Skin**:
    - **Gas gangrene**: benzylpenicillin and anti-toxin.
- see Fig. 1.11.

#### Clostridium tetani

- **Location**:
  - human and animal gastrointestinal tracts;
  - soil.
- **Transmission**: spores contaminate open wounds and produce an exotoxin (tetanospasmin).
- **Diseases**:
  - **Neurological**: tetanus (see Chapter 12, Nervous system infections)
- **Anti-microbial**:
  - **Neurological**:
    - **Tetanus**: human tetanus immunoglobulin.

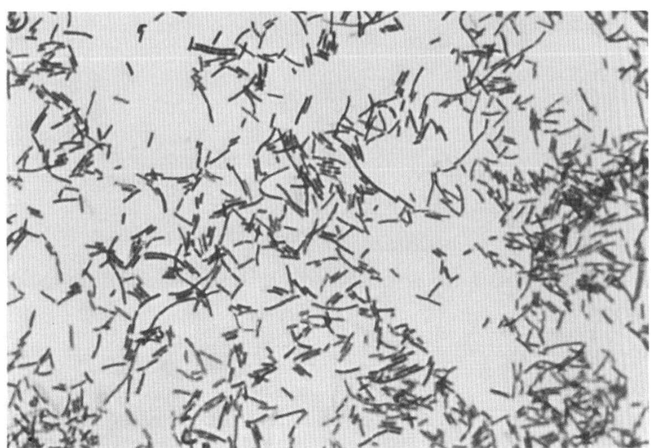

Fig. 1.11 *Clostridium perfringens* stained with Gram stain. Courtesy of the Academic Department of Infection & Immunity, University of Sheffield, UK.

- **Immunization (UK schedule)**: 2, 3 and 4 months, 3 years and 4 months, and 13–18 years old.
- See Fig. 1.12.

### Clostridium difficile

- **Location**: faecal commensal.
- **Transmission**: spores via faecal–oral route.
- **Diseases**:
  - **Gastrointestinal**: Pseudomembranous colitis (see Chapter 8, Gastrointestinal infections).
- **Treatment**:

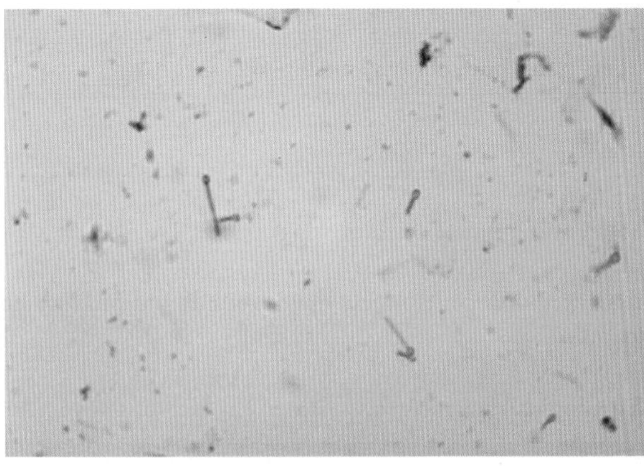

Fig. 1.12 *Clostridium tetani* stained with Gram stain. Courtesy of the Academic Department of Infection & Immunity, University of Sheffield, UK.

- **Gastrointestinal**:
  - **Pseudomembranous colitis**: discontinue causative antibiotic if possible and give metronidazole or vancomycin (severe or reinfection).

> **MICRO-facts**
>
> **Pseudomembranous colitis** is an exudative colitis, common after antibiotic therapy as normal gut flora is disrupted.

#### Clostridium botulinum

- **Location**: soil and plants.
- **Transmission**: Food ingestion (typically cans and jars, toxin formed preingestion) or wound contamination.
- **Diseases**:
  - **Neurological**: botulism (see Chapter 12, Nervous system infections).
- **Treatment**:
  - **Neurological**:
    - **Botulism**: botulism anti-toxin.

> **MICRO-facts**
>
> **Botox** is **bo**tulinum **tox**in and in addition to its use in **cosmetic surgery** it is also used clinically to treat **focal spasticity, blepharospasm** and **spasmodic torticollis.**

## 1.7 GRAM-NEGATIVE BACTERIA IDENTIFICATION FLOWCHART (FIG. 1.13)

## 1.8 GRAM-NEGATIVE BACTERIA

There are eight key Gram-negative (red staining) bacterial groups:

1. *Neisseria* spp.;
2. coliforms (also *Enterobacteriaceae*);
3. parvobacteria;
4. *Campylobacter* spp.;
5. *Helicobacter* spp.;
6. *Vibrio* spp.;
7. *Pseudomonas* spp.;
8. *Bartonella* spp.

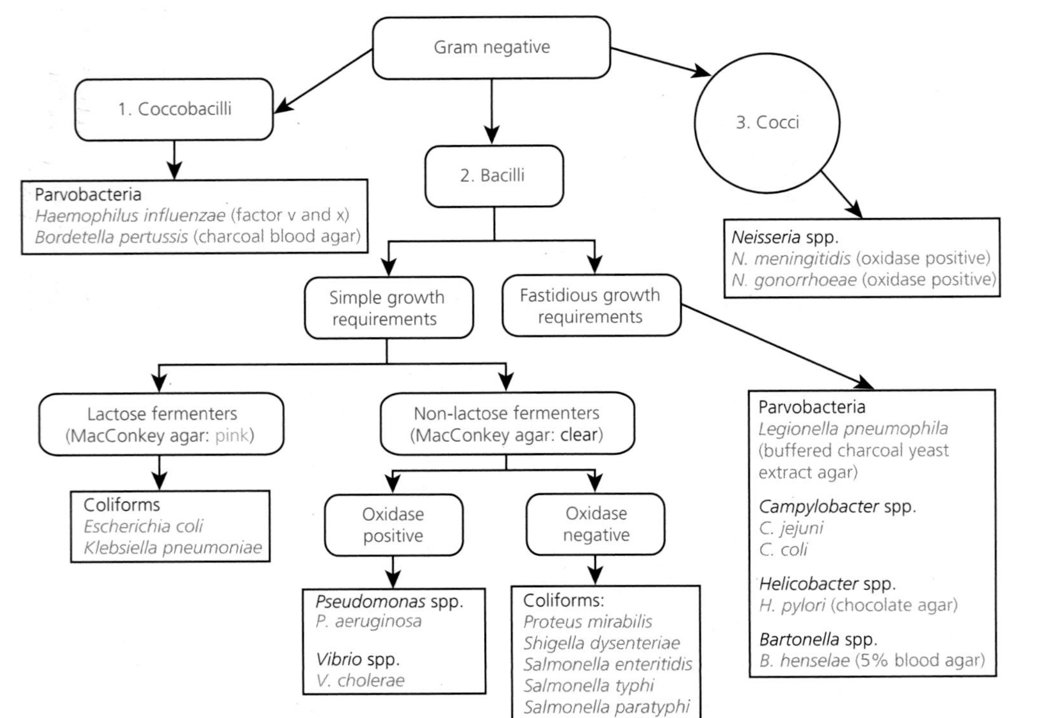


Fig. 1.13 **Gram-negative bacteria identification flowchart.**

## *NEISSERIA* SPP.

### Characteristics

- **Shape**: cocci in pairs (diplococci).
- **Characteristic morphology**: intracellular diplococci, commonly within neutrophils.
- **Staining**: Gram-negative.
- **Biochemical tests**:
    - **Oxidase test**: oxidase positive.
- **Oxygen requirement**: aerobic.

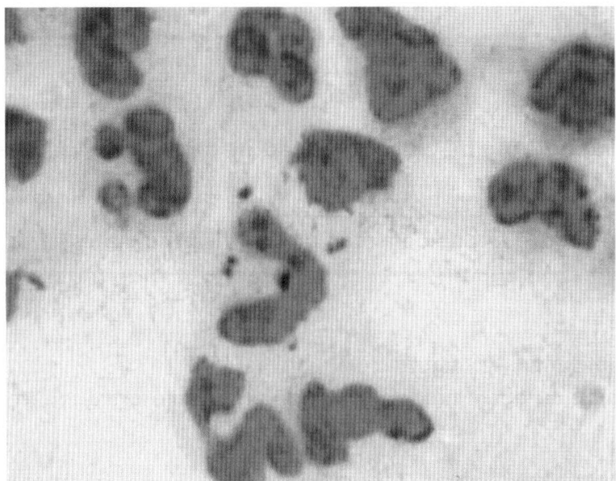

Fig. 1.14 *Neisseria meningitidis* stained with Gram stain. Courtesy of the Academic Department of Infection & Immunity, University of Sheffield, UK.

### Key examples

#### Neisseria meningitidis

> **MICRO-facts**
>
> **Meningococcal** disease is **life threatening** with severe complications – if suspected in the **community** give a **single dose of benzylpenicillin** (unless **strongly** penicillin allergic) and transfer to **hospital**.

- **Location**: nasopharynx in 5–20% of general population.
- **Transmission**: respiratory droplet spread or direct mucosal contact.
- **Diseases**:
    - **Neurological**: meningitis (see Chapter 12, Nervous system infections).

- **Blood**: septicaemia (with purpuric skin rash).
- **Anti-microbial**:
  - **Neurological**:
    - **Meningitis**: benzylpenicillin (community) or cefotaxime.
    - **Close contact prophylaxis**: rifampicin, ciprofloxacin or ceftriaxone.
  - **Blood**:
    - **Septicaemia**: benzylpenicillin (community) or cefotaxime.
  - **Immunization (UK schedule)**:
    - Group A and C strain available, group B currently unavailable.
    - **Meningococcal group C**: 3, 4 and 12 months.

**MICRO-print**

*NEISSERIA MENINGITIDIS*

***N. meningitidis*** can be further **grouped** by **capsular polysaccharides**:
**Group A**: most common in **sub-Saharan Africa.**
**Groups B and C**: most common serogroups in the **UK.**
**Group W135**: recent epidemics in many African countries.

### Neisseria gonorrhoeae

- **Location**: human genital tract.
- **Transmission**: direct mucosal contact (e.g. during sexual intercourse or birth).
- **Diseases**:
  - **Sexual health**: gonorrhoea.
  - **Ophthalmic**: ophthalmia neonatorum.
- **Anti-microbial**:
  - **Resistance**: penicillin resistance increasing.
  - **Sexual health**:
    - **Gonorrhoea**: ciprofloxacin or cefixime (see Chapter 11, Genitourinary infections).
    - **Pelvic inflammatory disease**: doxycycline and metronidazole and ceftriaxone or ofloxacin and metronidazole.
  - **Ophthalmic**:
    - **Ophthalmia neonatorum**: ceftriaxone or cefotaxime (see Chapter 15, Congenital, neonatal and childhood infections).

**MICRO-facts**

Ophthalmia neonatorum is a notifiable disease in the UK.

## COLIFORMS (*ENTEROBACTERIACEAE*)

### Characteristics

- **Shape**: bacilli.
- **Staining**: Gram-negative.
- **Culture techniques**:
  - **MacConkey agar**:
    - **Red/pink colony**: *Escherichia* spp. and *Klebsiella* spp.
    - **Clear colony**: *Salmonella* spp., *Shigella* spp. and *Proteus* spp.
- **Oxygen requirement**: aerobic.

### Key examples

#### Escherichia coli

- **Location**: intestinal tract commensal.
- **Transmission**: faecal–oral (e.g. undercooked meat) or local spread of faecal flora (e.g. UTI).
- **Diseases**:
  - **Gastrointestinal**: gastroenteritis and peritonitis (see Chapter 8, Gastrointestinal infections).
  - **Urinary tract**: UTI (see Chapter 11, Genitourinary infections).
  - **Respiratory**: pneumonia (hospital acquired and neonatal) (see Chapter 7, Respiratory infections).
  - **Neurological**: meningitis (neonatal) (see Chapter 12, Nervous system infections).
  - **Blood**: septicaemia.
  - **Skin**: wound infection (see Chapter 13, Skin infections).
  - **Systemic**: haemolytic uraemic syndrome (HUS) (haemolytic anaemia, thrombocytopenia and acute renal failure).
- **Anti-microbial**:
  - **Resistance**: penicillins and cephalosporins (extended spectrum B-lactamases (ESBLs)).
  - **Gastrointestinal**:
    - **Gastroenteritis**: self-limiting disease.
  - **Urinary tract**:
    - **UTI**: trimethoprim or nitrofurantoin.
  - **Respiratory**:
    - **Pneumonia**: co-amoxiclav or cefuroxime or ciprofloxacin.
  - **Neurological**:
    - **Meningitis**: cefotaxime.
  - **Blood**:
    - **Septicaemia**: amoxicillin or second/third-generation cephalosporin (e.g. cefuroxime).
  - **Skin**:
    - **Wound infection**: amoxicillin or second/third-generation cephalosporin (e.g. cefuroxime).

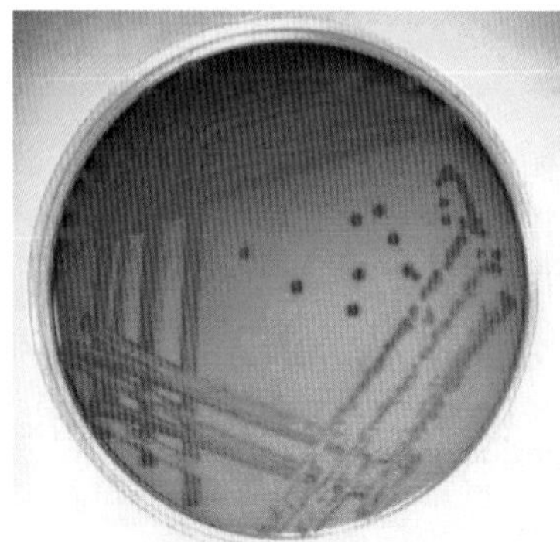

Fig. 1.15 *Escherichia coli* on MacConkey agar. Courtesy of the Academic Department of Infection & Immunity, University of Sheffield, UK.

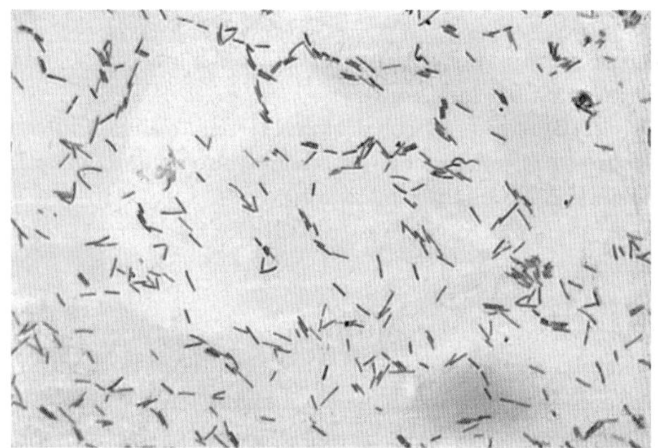

Fig. 1.16 *Escherichia coli* stained with Gram stain. Courtesy of the Academic Department of Infection & Immunity, University of Sheffield, UK.

## MICRO-facts

***Escherichia coli*** subtypes:

**Enterotoxigenic** (ETEC): **watery** diarrhoea, very common cause of traveller's diarrhoea.

**Enteroinvasive** (EIEC): ***Shigella***-esque gastroenteritis.

**Enterohaemorrhagic (EHEC)**: commonest serotype is **O157**:**H7**, causes **bloody** diarrhoea and **HUS**.

*Salmonella enteritidis* (*also Salmonella enterica*)

- **Location**: commensal of animal gastrointestinal tracts.
- **Transmission**: faecal–oral.
- **Diseases**:
  - **Gastrointestinal**: gastroenteritis (food borne) (see Chapter 8, Gastrointestinal infections).
  - **Blood**: bacteraemia (uncommon complication of gastroenteritis).
  - **Post-infective**: reactive arthritis.
- **Treatment**:
  - **Gastrointestinal**:
    - **Gastroenteritis**: self-limiting disease.

**MICRO-print**

***SALMONELLA TYPHI*** **AND** ***SALMONELLA PARATYPHI*** **(TYPES A, B AND C)**

**Location:** human colon, not found in animals.
**Transmission:** faecal–oral.
**Diseases:**
**Gastrointestinal:** typhoid and paratyphoid (enteric fever).
**Post-infective:** reactive arthritis.
**Treatment:**
**Gastrointestinal:**
**Typhoid and paratyphoid:** ciprofloxacin.

***KLEBSIELLA PNEUMONIAE***

**Location:** human gastrointestinal and upper respiratory tracts.
**Transmission:** respiratory droplets or local spread of faecal flora.
**Diseases:**
**Respiratory:** pneumonia (hospital acquired).
**Urinary tract:** urinary tract infection.
**Neurological:** meningitis (neonatal, rare).
**Blood:** septicaemia.
**Anti-microbial:**
**Respiratory:**
**Pneumonia:** cefuroxime or ciprofloxacin.
**Urinary tract:**
**Urinary tract infection:** trimethoprim or nitrofurantoin or an oral cephalosporin.

***PROTEUS MIRABILIS***

**Location:** soil, water and human gastrointestinal tract.
**Transmission:** local spread of faecal flora.
**Diseases:**
**Urinary tract:** urinary tract infection.
**Anti-microbial:**

*continued...*

continued...

**Urinary tract:**
**Urinary tract infection:** trimethoprim or nitrofurantoin.

***SHIGELLA DYSENTERIAE***
**Location:** human gastrointestinal tract.
**Transmission:** faecal–oral.
**Diseases:**
**Gastrointestinal:** bacillary dysentery (with mucus and blood).
**Post-infective:** reactive arthritis.
**Anti-microbial:**
**Gastrointestinal:**
**Gastroenteritis:** ciprofloxacin or azithromycin.

## PARVOBACTERIA

### Characteristics

- **Shape**: bacilli except for *H. influenzae* (coccobacilli).
- **Characteristic morphology**: small cells.
- **Staining**: Gram-negative.
- **Culture techniques**:
    - **Factor V and X discs**: *H. influenzae.*
    - **Charcoal blood agar**: *B. pertussis.*
    - **Buffered charcoal yeast extract agar**: *Legionella pneumophila.*
- **Oxygen requirement**: aerobic.

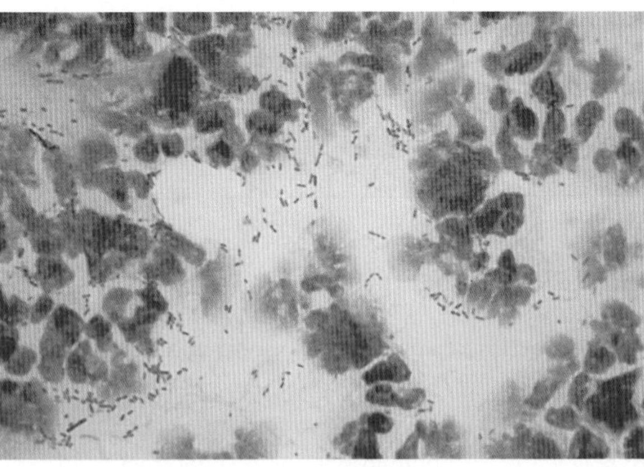

Fig. 1.17 *Haemophilus influenzae* in cerebrospinal fluid, stained with Gram stain. Courtesy of the Academic Department of Infection & Immunity, University of Sheffield, UK.

## Key examples

### Haemophilus influenzae

- **Shape**: coccobacilli.
- **Location**: both the capsulated and non-capsulated forms can be upper respiratory tract commensals.
- **Transmission**: respiratory droplet spread.
- **Diseases**:
  - **Respiratory**: acute epiglottitis and pneumonia (community acquired) (see Chapter 7, Respiratory infections).
  - **Neurological**: meningitis (see Chapter 12, Nervous system infections).
  - **Skin**: cellulitis (see Chapter 13, Skin infections).
  - **ENT**: otitis media (see Chapter 7, Respiratory infections).
  - **Bones and joints**: osteomyelitis and septic arthritis (see Chapter 14, Bone and joint infections).
- **Anti-microbial**:
  - **Resistance**: amoxicillin, erythromycin and co-amoxiclav.
  - **Respiratory**:
    - **Acute epiglottitis**: cefotaxime or chloramphenicol.
    - **Pneumonia**: amoxicillin or benzylpenicillin (previously healthy chest) or erythromycin (penicillin allergy).
  - **Neurological**:
    - **Meningitis**: cefotaxime or chloramphenicol (penicillin or cephalosporin hypersensitivity or cefotaxime resistance).
    - **Close contact prophylaxis**: rifampicin.
  - **Skin**:
    - **Cellulitis**: cefotaxime.
  - **ENT**:
    - **Otitis media**: amoxicillin or erythromycin (penicillin allergy) (many cases resolve without treatment; use antibiotics if no improvement after 72 hours, systemic features, high risk of complications or mastoiditis present).
  - **Bones and joints**:
    - **Osteomyelitis**: cefotaxime.
    - **Septic arthritis**: cefotaxime.
  - **Immunization (UK schedule)**: 2, 3, 4 and 12 months.

> **MICRO-facts**
>
> There are **six serotypes** of ***Haemophilus influenzae***, serotype **b** (**capsulated**) is the most **pathogenic** but it is **rare** in the **UK** due to **immunization.**

### Bordetella pertussis

- **Shape**: bacilli.
- **Location**: human respiratory tract.
- **Transmission**: respiratory droplet spread.
- **Diseases**:
  - **Respiratory**: whooping cough (pertussis) (see Chapter 7, Respiratory infections).
- **Anti-microbial**:
  - **Respiratory**:
    - **Whooping cough**: erythromycin.
    - **Close contact prophylaxis**: erythromycin (non-immune or partially immune patients).
  - **Immunization (UK schedule)**: 2, 3 and 4 months, and 3 years and 4 months.

> **MICRO-facts**
>
> The **pertussis cough** is characterized by an **inspiratory 'whoop'** sound.

### Legionella pneumophila

- **Shape**: bacilli.
- **Location**: warm water (e.g. air-conditioning units and hot water tanks).
- **Transmission**: inhalation of aerosolized droplet.
- **Diseases**:
  - **Respiratory**: Legionnaires' disease (severe atypical pneumonia).
- **Anti-microbial**:
  - **Respiratory**:
    - **Legionnaires' disease**: clarithromycin (with ciprofloxacin and/or rifampicin in severe cases).

> **MICRO-print**
>
> *LEGIONELLA PNEUMOPHILA*
>
> ***L. pneumophila*** also causes **Pontiac fever**, which is similar to **legionella without lower respiratory tract** involvement.

## *CAMPYLOBACTER* SPP.

> **MICRO-facts**
>
> *Campylobacter* spp. are the commonest cause of diarrhoea in the UK.

### Characteristics

- **Shape**: curved bacilli.
- **Characteristic morphology**: colourless or grey colonies.
- **Staining**: Gram-negative.
- **Oxygen requirement**: microaerophilic (optimal growth at 5% oxygen).

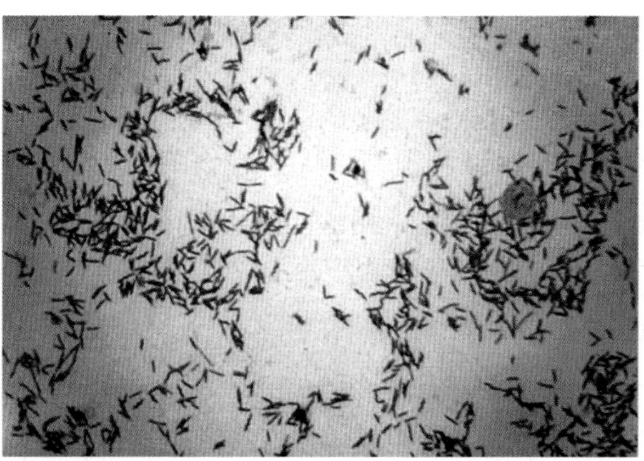

Fig. 1.18 *Campylobacter jejuni* stained with Gram stain. Courtesy of the Academic Department of Infection & Immunity, University of Sheffield, UK.

### Key example

#### Campylobacter jejuni *and* Campylobacter coli

- **Location**: human and animal gastrointestinal tracts.
- **Transmission**: faecal–oral route from contaminated poultry (*C. jejuni*) or pig meat (*C. coli*) or unpasteurized milk.
- **Diseases**:
  - **Gastrointestinal**: gastroenteritis (see Chapter 8, Gastrointestinal infections).
  - **Blood**: septicaemia (rare).
  - **Post-infective**: Guillain–Barré syndrome(1–2 weeks post infection).
- **Anti-microbial**:
  - **Gastrointestinal**:
    - **Gastroenteritis**: usually self-limiting, ciprofloxacin or erythromycin (severe cases).

## *HELICOBACTER* SPP.

### Characteristics

- **Shape**: curved bacilli.
- **Staining**: Gram-negative.

- **Biochemical tests**:
  - **Urease tests ($^{13}$C urea breath test and rapid urease test)**: positive.
- **Culture techniques**:
  - **Chocolate agar**: *H. pylori.*
- **Serological tests**: antibodies can be detected in the blood and stool.
- **Oxygen requirement**: aerobic.

### Key example

#### Helicobacter pylori

- **Location**: human gastric mucosa.
- **Transmission**: faecal–oral.
- **Diseases**:
  - **Gastrointestinal**: chronic gastritis, duodenal and gastric ulcers and risk factor for gastric cancer.
- **Anti-microbial**:
  - **Gastrointestinal**: clarithromycin and amoxicillin or metronidazole.

> **MICRO-facts**
>
> ***Helicobacter pylori*** has been shown to **increase** the **risk** of **duodenal ulcers.**
>
> **Triple therapies** are used to **eradicate *Helicobacter pylori*** and they include a combination of **antibiotics** with a **proton pump inhibitor** (e.g. omeprazole).

## *VIBRIO* SPP.

### Characteristics

- **Shape**: vibrio (comma shaped).
- **Staining**: Gram-negative.
- **Biochemical tests**:
  - **Oxidase test**: oxidase positive.
- **Oxygen requirement**: aerobic.

### Key example

#### Vibrio cholerae

- **Location**: water and seafood.
- **Transmission**: faecal–oral and consumption of infected seafood.
- **Diseases**:
  - **Gastrointestinal**: cholera (see Chapter 8, Gastrointestinal infections).
- **Anti-microbial**:

- **Gastrointestinal**:
  - **Cholera**: ciprofloxacin (severe cases).

**MICRO-facts**

***Vibrio cholerae*** causes a significant **secretory diarrhoea** with up to **25 litres** lost per day – **rehydration** is essential!

**MICRO-print**

***VIBRIO CHOLERAE***

There are over **139 serogroups** of ***Vibrio cholerae*****. Epidemics** are generally caused by **serogroup O1**, of which there are **two biotypes: El-Tor** (named after an area in Egypt where it was discovered); **classic**.

However, it is now accepted that non-O1 vibrios can also cause epidemics.

## *PSEUDOMONAS* SPP.

### Characteristics

- **Shape**: bacilli.
- **Characteristic morphology**: produces a blue-green pigment (pyocyanin) when grown on normal agar.
- **Staining**: Gram-negative.
- **Biochemical tests**:
  - **Oxidase test**: oxidase positive.
- **Culture techniques**:
  - **MacConkey agar**: clear colony.
- **Oxygen requirement**: aerobic.

### Key example

#### Pseudomonas aeruginosa

- **Location**: moist environments, skin, respiratory and gastrointestinal tracts.
- **Transmission**: inhalation of aerosolized droplet and faecal contamination.
- **Diseases**:
  - Tends to cause disease in patients with multiple co-morbidities or severe illness (e.g. patients on ICU).
  - **Respiratory**: pneumonia (hospital acquired and patients with cystic fibrosis, bronchiectasis and artificial ventilation) (see Chapter 7, Respiratory infections).

- **Urinary tract**: UTI (long-term catheterization) (see Chapter 11, Genitourinary infections).
- **Blood**: septicaemia.
- **Ophthalmic**: bacterial keratitis.
- **Skin**: wound, burn and IV catheter infections (see Chapter 13, Skin infections).
- **ENT**: otitis externa (see Chapter 7, Respiratory infections).
- **Cardiovascular**: infective endocarditis (see Chapter 9, Cardiovascular infections).

- **Anti-microbial**:
  - **Respiratory**:
    - **Pneumonia**: ceftazidime or piperacillin with tazobactam or ciprofloxacin.
  - **Urinary tract**:
    - **UTI**: ceftazidime.
  - **Blood**:
    - **Septicaemia**: piperacillin with tazobactam or ceftazidime or imipenem with cilastatin or meropenem and an aminoglycoside (e.g. gentamicin).
  - **ENT**:
    - **Otitis externa**: ciprofloxacin or an aminoglycoside.

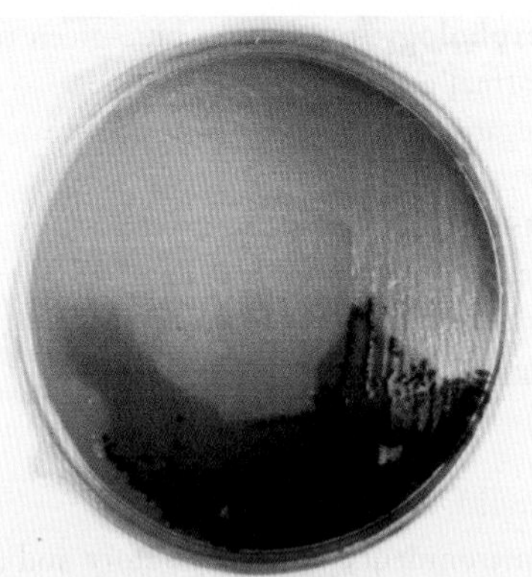

Fig. 1.19 *Pseudomonas aeruginosa* showing oxidase positive test. Courtesy of the Academic Department of Infection & Immunity, University of Sheffield, UK.

## BARTONELLA SPP.

### Characteristics

- **Shape**: bacilli.
- **Staining**: Gram-negative.

- **Oxygen requirement**: aerobic.

### Key example

#### Bartonella henselae

- **Location**: oral commensal of cats.
- **Transmission**: scratch or bite from cat.
- **Diseases**: cat scratch fever (papule at site of scratch, regional lymphadenopathy with granulomatous lesions develops 1–2 weeks later, resolves over 2 months).
- **Anti-microbial**:
  - **Cat scratch fever**: uncomplicated cases do not require treatment, complications may be treated with erythromycin or doxycycline (clinical efficacy has not been proven).

> **MICRO-facts**
>
> In immunocompromised states, cat scratch fever can cause encephalopathy, granulomatous hepatitis, endocarditis and osteomyelitis.

## 1.9 POOR/NON-GRAM-STAINING BACTERIA IDENTIFICATION FLOWCHART

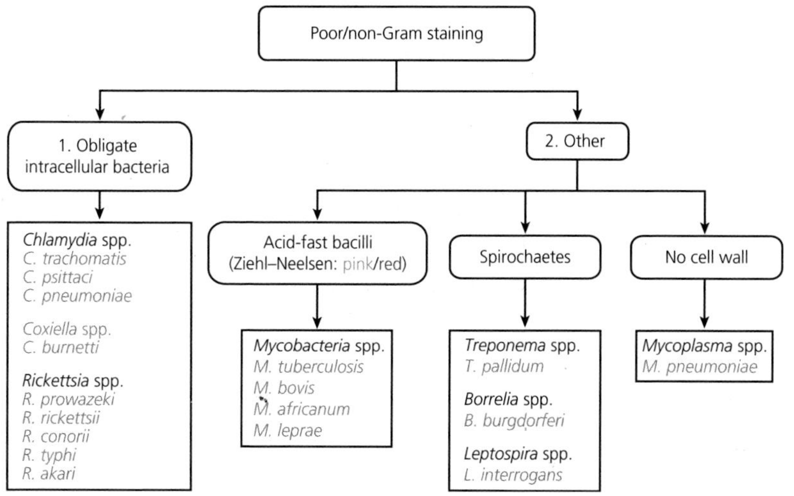


Fig. 1.20 Poor/non-Gram-staining bacteria identification flowchart.

# 1.10 POOR/NON-GRAM-STAINING BACTERIA

There are eight key bacterial groups that either stain poorly or not at all with the Gram stain:

1. *Chlamydia* spp.;
2. *Mycobacterium* spp.;
3. *Treponema* spp.;
4. *Mycoplasma* spp.;
5. *Rickettsia* spp.;
6. *Leptospira* spp.;
7. *Coxiella* spp.;
8. *Borrelia* spp.

## *CHLAMYDIA* SPP.

**MICRO-print**

***CHLAMYDIA* SPP.**

*Chlamydia* spp. exist in two forms:

**Elementary body**: extracellular form, able to withstand harmful environments and infect cells.

**Reticulate body**: intracellular form, replicate after infection.

### Characteristics

- **Shape**: no distinct bacterial shape.
- **Characteristic morphology**:
    - Intracellular growth.
    - **Light microscopy**: cytoplasmic inclusions visible.
- **Serological tests**:
    - **ELISA or immunofluorescence**: detects chlamydial antigens in urine or exudates.
- **Nucleic acid techniques**:
    - **PCR assay**: detects bacterial DNA in urine.

### Key example

Chlamydia trachomatis

**MICRO-facts**

**Trachoma** is a **preventable** cause of **blindness** that is caused by **multiple *Chlamydia trachomatis* infections**.

- **Location**: human genital tract and eyes.
- **Transmission**: direct mucosal contact or skin contact (e.g. trachoma).
- **Diseases**:
  - **Sexual health**: chlamydia, pelvic inflammatory disease and epididymitis (see Chapter 11, Genitourinary infections).
  - **Ophthalmic**: ophthalmia neonatorum and trachoma (see Chapter 15, Congenital, neonatal and childhood infections).
  - **Post-infective**: reactive arthritis (including Reiter's syndrome).
- **Anti-microbial**:
  - **Sexual health**:
    - **Chlamydia**: doxycycline or azithromycin or erythromycin (pregnancy).
    - **Pelvic inflammatory disease**: doxycycline and metronidazole and ceftriaxone or ofloxacin and metronidazole.
  - **Ophthalmic**:
    - **Ophthalmia neonatorum**: erythromycin.
    - **Trachoma**: azithromycin.

**MICRO-print**

*CHLAMYDOPHILA PSITTACI*

**Location**: birds.
**Transmission**: inhalation of infected material, especially dried faeces.
**Diseases**:
**Respiratory**: psittacosis (an atypical pneumonia also known as parrot disease).
**Anti-microbial**:
**Respiratory**:
**Psittacosis**: tetracycline.

*CHLAMYDOPHILA PNEUMONIAE*

**Location**: human respiratory tract.
**Transmission**: respiratory droplet spread.
**Diseases**:
**Respiratory**: pneumonia (atypical), pharyngitis and sinusitis.
**Anti-microbial**:
**Respiratory**:
**Pneumonia**: erythromycin or tetracycline.

## *MYCOBACTERIA* SPP.

### Characteristics

- **Shape**: bacilli.
- **Characteristic morphology**: intracellular within macrophages.

- **Staining**:
  - acid-fast bacilli (Ziehl–Neelsen staining: pink/red);
  - auramine–rhodamine stain (bright yellow with fluorescence microscopy).
- **Culture techniques**:
  - Lowenstein–Jensen culture medium (up to 12 weeks);
  - rapid liquid culture (allows identification within 7–14 days).
- **Nucleic acid techniques**: PCR techniques allow rapid identification.
- **Oxygen requirement**: obligate aerobe.

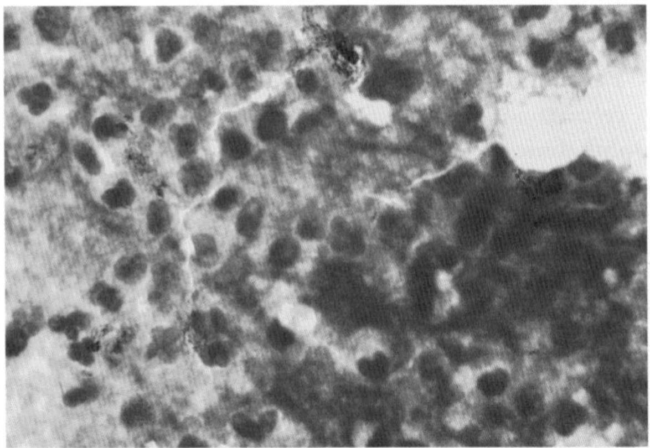

Fig. 1.21 *Mycobacterium tuberculosis* in a sputum sample stained with Ziehl–Neelsen stain. Courtesy of the Academic Department of Infection & Immunity, University of Sheffield, UK.

## Key examples

### Mycobacterium tuberculosis/africanum/bovis

- **Location**: human (*M. tuberculosis*) and cow (*M. bovis*) reservoir.
- **Transmission**: respiratory droplet spread and ingestion of contaminated milk (*M. bovis*).
- **Diseases**: tuberculosis (TB) (see Chapter 7, Respiratory infections).
- **Anti-microbial**:
  - **Resistance**: multiple strains of *Mycobacteria* spp. are now resistant to traditional anti-TB drugs (multiple drug-resistant TB (MDR) and extremely drug-resistant TB (XDR)).
  - **Tuberculosis**:
    - **Initial phase**: rifampicin and isoniazid with ethambutol and pyrazinamide (2 months).
    - **Continuation phase**: rifampicin and isoniazid (4 months).

### Mycobacterium leprae

- **Location**: human only reservoir.
- **Transmission**: respiratory droplet spread.
- **Diseases**: leprosy.
- **Anti-microbial**:
  - **Leprosy**: rifampicin and dapsone and clofazimine.

> **MICRO-facts**
>
> **Leprosy** is characterized by:
>
> **Skin lesions**: hypopigmented with reduced sensation.
>
> **Nerve lesions**: thickened and peripheral neuropathy.
>
> **Eye lesions**: blindness.

## *TREPONEMA* SPP.

### Characteristics

- **Shape**: spirochaete.
- **Characteristic morphology**:
  - **Dark field microscopy**: spirochaetes are visible only under dark field microscopy.
- **Serological tests**:
  - **Agglutination**:
    - **Venereal Disease Research Laboratory (VDRL) test or rapid plasma reagent (RPR) test**: infection with *Treponema pallidum* results in the production of antibodies to human lipids released during bacterial damage (also bacterial lipids). The addition of an extract of beef heart (cardiolipin) to a serum sample results in agglutination.
    - ***T. pallidum* particle agglutination (TPPA) test**: gelatin particles are coated with *T. pallidum* antigen and then added to the sample serum.
    - ***T. pallidum* haemagglutination (TPHA) test**: red blood cells are presensitized to *T. pallidum* antigen and then exposed to the sample serum.
  - **ELISA**: detection of *T. pallidum* IgG or IgM antibodies.
  - **Immunofluorescence**:
    - **Fluorescent treponemal antibody absorption (FTA-ABS)**: cross-reacting antibodies are removed before testing to increase specificity.

### Key example

#### Treponema pallidum

- **Location**: human genital tract.
- **Transmission**: direct mucosal contact (especially during sexual intercourse), *in utero* or perinatally.
- **Diseases**:
  - **Sexual health**: syphilis (see Chapter 11, Genitourinary infections).
- **Anti-microbial**:
  - **Syphilis**: benzathine penicillin or doxycycline or erythromycin.

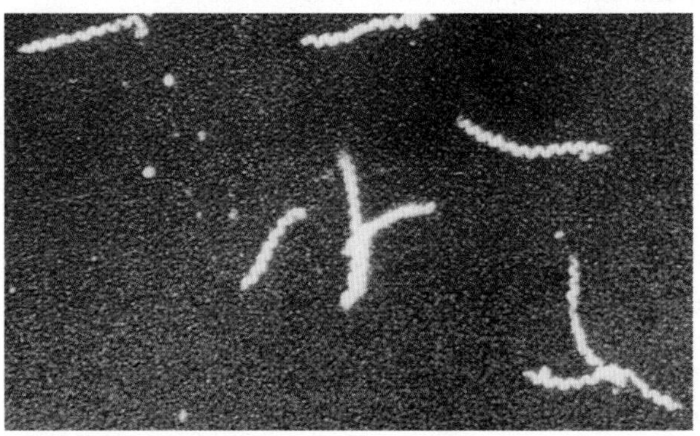

Fig. 1.22 *Treponema pallidum* shown under dark field microscopy. Courtesy of the Academic Department of Infection & Immunity, University of Sheffield, UK.

## *MYCOPLASMA* SPP.

### Characteristics

- **Shape**: bacilli.
- **Characteristic morphology**: very small organism without a cell wall.

### Key example

#### Mycoplasma pneumoniae

- **Location**: human respiratory tract.
- **Transmission**: respiratory droplet spread.
- **Diseases**:
  - **Respiratory**: pneumonia (atypical and community acquired) (see Chapter 7, Respiratory infections).
- **Anti-microbial**:
  - **Respiratory**:
    - **Pneumonia**: erythromycin or tetracycline.

## MICRO-print

### *RICKETTSIA* SPP.

Characteristics

**Shape**: bacilli.

**Characteristic morphology**: small and intracellular.

**Serological tests**:

**ELISA (enzyme-linked immunosorbent assay) test**: detects antibody.

Key examples

***Rickettsia prowazeki/rickettsii/conorii/typhi/akari:***

**Location**: arthropods and rodents (dependent on species).

**Transmission**: arthropod bites (e.g. ticks).

**Diseases**:

**Rocky mountain spotted fever** (principally *R. rickettsii*);
**typhus** (multiple forms depending on *Rickettsia* species).

**Anti-microbial**: doxycycline or chloramphenicol or tetracycline.

### *LEPTOSPIRA* SPP.

Characteristics

**Shape**: spirochaete.

**Staining**: Gram-negative.

**Oxygen requirements**: aerobic.

Key example

***Leptospira interrogans:***

**Location**: water (e.g. pools, canals and rivers) and animals (e.g. rats).

**Transmission**: exposure of open wounds, mucous membranes or conjunctivae to infected material (e.g. rat urine).

**Diseases**: leptospirosis (Weil's disease) (broad spectrum of severity from flu-like symptoms to multisystem infection).

**Anti-microbial**:

**Leptospirosis**: doxycycline or benzylpenicillin or amoxicillin.

### *COXIELLA* SPP.

Characteristics

**Shape**: bacilli.

**Characteristic morphology**: small and intracellular within macrophages.

Key example

***Coxiella burnetii:***

**Location**: cattle, sheep and soil.

**Transmission**: inhalation of airborne particles (e.g. urine or faeces) or arthropod bites (e.g. ticks).

**Diseases**:

**Respiratory**: Q-fever (atypical pneumonia).

**Cardiovascular**: endocarditis.

**Anti-microbial**: tetracycline or doxycycline.

*continued...*

*continued...*

***BORRELIA* SPP.**

Characteristics

**Shape**: spirochaete.

**Oxygen requirements**: anaerobic or microaerophilic.

Key example

***Borrelia burgdorferi:***

**Location**: mice.

**Transmission**: ixodid tick bites (commonly in forested areas).

**Diseases**: Lyme disease.

**Anti-microbial**:

**Lyme disease**: doxycycline or amoxicillin.

# 2 Viruses

## 2.1 VIRAL STRUCTURE

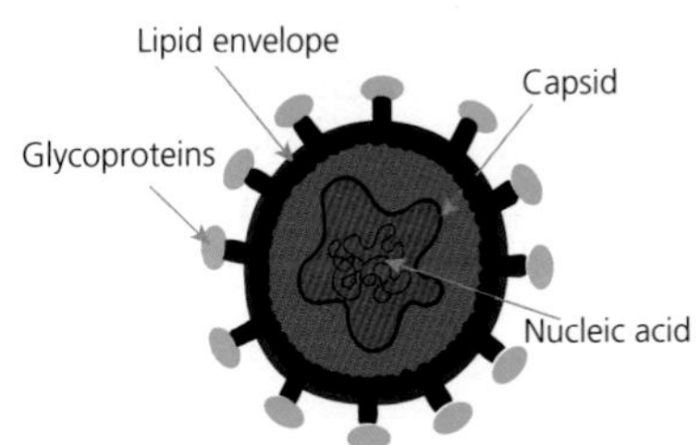


Fig. 2.1 Generic viral structure.

### LIPID ENVELOPE

- Usually formed from a lipid bilayer taken from their host, into which the virus inserts its own glycoproteins (enveloped virus).
- Not all viruses have envelopes (naked virus).
- Viruses without envelopes are less prone to damage by external factors, such as pH, than those with envelopes.
- The lipid envelope also determines how viruses enter their host cells.

### GLYCOPROTEINS

- Either function as transport channels or form viral antigens

### CAPSID

- Capsids are proteins that form a coat around the nucleic acid.
- The capsid and genetic information are grouped together and are collectively known as the nucleocapsid.
- Often the whole virus is actually just a nucleocapsid, without a membrane or envelope.

### GENETIC MATERIAL

- The genetic material within viruses can be single- or double-stranded deoxyribonucleic acid (DNA) or ribonucleic acid (RNA).
- A protein coating often protects the genome from external factors.

## 2.2 VIRAL INFECTION AND REPLICATION

### ADSORPTION

- Glycoproteins in the viral lipid envelope or molecules on the nucleocapsid (naked viruses) attach to specific receptor molecules on the host cell.
- This viral–host receptor molecule relationship is often highly specific. Accordingly, many viruses can only infect a limited range of cells.
- For example, the human immunodeficiency virus (HIV) preferentially infects T-helper cells as they express CD4 and CXCR4 receptor molecules on their cell membrane. The glycoprotein 120 molecule found in the lipid envelope of the HIV is able to bind with these receptor molecules.

### ENTRY

- The mechanism by which viruses gain entry to their host cells is dependent upon their structure; in particular, whether a lipid membrane is present.
  - **Enveloped virus**:
    - **Cytoplasmic membrane fusion**: the virus fuses with the host cell cytoplasmic membrane and the viral contents are then released into the cytoplasm.
    - **Endocytosis**: the virus is engulfed by the host cell cytoplasmic membrane.
  - **Naked virus**:
    - **Direct**: the virus passes directly across the host cell cytoplasmic membrane.
    - **Endocytosis**.

### UNCOATING

- Once inside the host cell, the viral lipid envelope or capsid is shed and the viral nucleic acids are released.
- At this stage, the virus ceases to be infective and will only regain infectivity after new virions have been formed (eclipse phase).

### REPLICATION

- Viral replication is broadly a two-stage process; both viral proteins and nucleic acid must be replicated to form new virus particles.

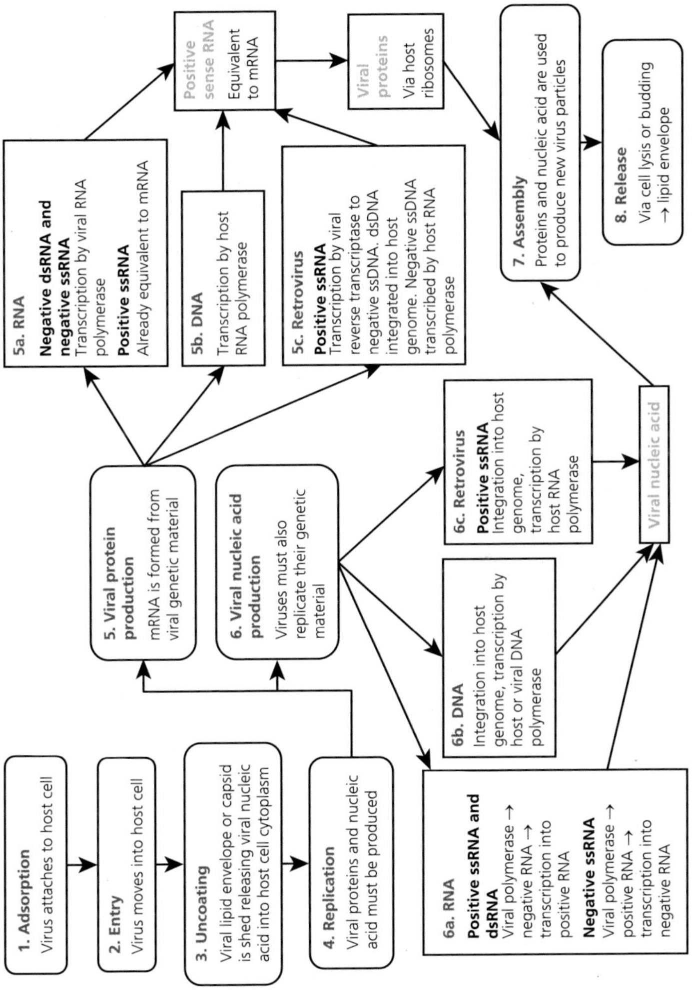

**1. Adsorption**
Virus attaches to host cell

**2. Entry**
Virus moves into host cell

**3. Uncoating**
Viral lipid envelope or capsid is shed releasing viral nucleic acid into host cell cytoplasm

**4. Replication**
Viral proteins and nucleic acid must be produced

**5. Viral protein production**
mRNA is formed from viral genetic material

**6. Viral nucleic acid production**
Viruses must also replicate their genetic material

**5a. RNA**
**Negative dsRNA and negative ssRNA**
Transcription by viral RNA polymerase
**Positive ssRNA**
Already equivalent to mRNA

**5b. DNA**
Transcription by host RNA polymerase

**5c. Retrovirus**
**Positive ssRNA**
Transcription by viral reverse transcriptase to negative ssDNA. dsDNA integrated into host genome. Negative ssDNA transcribed by host RNA polymerase

Positive sense RNA
Equivalent to mRNA

Viral proteins
Via host ribosomes

**6a. RNA**
**Positive ssRNA and dsRNA**
Viral polymerase → negative RNA → transcription into positive RNA
**Negative ssRNA**
Viral polymerase → positive RNA → transcription into negative RNA

**6b. DNA**
Integration into host genome, transcription by host or viral DNA polymerase

**6c. Retrovirus**
**Positive ssRNA**
Integration into host genome, transcription by host RNA polymerase

Viral nucleic acid

**7. Assembly**
Proteins and nucleic acid are used to produce new virus particles

**8. Release**
Via cell lysis or budding → lipid envelope

Fig. 2.2 Viral infection and replication flowchart.

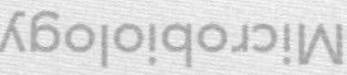

## VIRAL PROTEIN PRODUCTION

- Viruses must first transcribe their genetic material into messenger RNA (mRNA) in order to use host ribosomes to produce new viral proteins.
- This process varies depending on the form and sense of the viral genetic material.
  - **Forms**:
    - **RNA**: single-stranded (ssRNA) or double-stranded (dsRNA).
    - **DNA**: double-stranded (dsDNA).
  - **Sense**:
    - **Sense (positive sense, +ve)**: genetic material is ready for translation, and is already equivalent to mRNA.
    - **Anti-sense (negative sense, –ve)**: genetic material requires transcription to mRNA before translation can occur.
- **RNA**:
  - **–ve dsRNA and –ve ssRNA**: use viral RNA polymerase to form +ve ssRNA, which is equivalent to mRNA.
  - **+ve ssRNA**: already equivalent to mRNA.
- **DNA**:
  - DNA viruses have the equivalent of a positive and negative sense single strand.
  - They use host cell RNA polymerase to transcribe the negative sense strand into +ve ssRNA, which is equivalent to mRNA.
- **Retroviruses**:
  - retroviruses contain +ve ssRNA;
  - this is transcribed by viral reverse transcriptase into –ve ssRNA;
  - this is then used to form dsDNA, which is integrated into the host genome;
  - the negative sense strand is then transcribed by the host RNA polymerase to form mRNA (similar to the DNA process);
  - after mRNA or the +ve ssRNA has been formed, the host cell ribosomes are used as a site of viral protein synthesis.

## VIRAL NUCLEIC ACID PRODUCTION

- The mechanism of this process is also determined by the form and sense of the viral genetic material.
- **RNA**:
  - **+ve ssRNA and dsRNA**: viral polymerase produces multiple –ve ssRNA, which is transcribed into +ve ssRNA. With dsRNA, only the negative sense strand is converted into +ve ssRNA.
  - **–ve ssRNA**: the inverse of the above process – viral polymerase produces multiple +ve ssRNA, which is then transcribed into –ve ssRNA.

- **DNA**:
    - The viral genetic material is transcribed by viral DNA polymerase and then incorporated into the host genome.
    - Host or viral DNA polymerase is then used to produce multiple viral genetic material.
- **Retroviruses**:
    - Following integration into the host genome by viral reverse transcriptase, host RNA polymerase transcribes the viral DNA into RNA.

### ASSEMBLY

- Viral progeny are formed by integrating the new viral proteins and genetic material.

### RELEASE

- Viruses are released from their host cell either by host cell lysis or by a process called budding, in which the virus forms an envelope from the host cell cytoplasmic membrane.

## 2.3 DIAGNOSIS OF VIRAL INFECTIONS

There are two broad approaches to detecting and diagnosing a viral infection in the laboratory: **viral detection** and **host response**.

### VIRAL DETECTION

#### Cell culture

- Viruses must be cultured in medium that contains living cells such as monkey kidney.
- Viral growth can be identified by observing:
    - **Cytopathic effect**: a characteristic cellular change due to viral growth (e.g. respiratory syncytial virus (RSV) culture leads to multinucleated giant cells).
    - **Haemadsorption**: the envelope protein haemagglutinin (HA) causes added red blood cells to attach to the viral infected cell. Examples include influenza and mumps virus.
    - **Viral antibody**: a positive response to the addition of viral antibody is detected by a range of methods, including enzyme-linked immunosorbent assay (ELISA) and immunofluorescence.

#### Microscopic techniques

- **Light microscopy**: detects inclusion bodies (collections of viral particles) within the infected cell. Some have a characteristic appearance such as Negri bodies with rabies infection.

- **Electron microscopy**: detects viruses and viral particles.

### Viral antigen detection

- **ELISA and immunofluorescence**: see Chapter 1, Bacteria for further details.

### Viral nucleic acid

- The sequencing of viral nucleic acids has enabled the creation of highly sensitive diagnostic tests.
- A complementary DNA or RNA probe to the viral nucleic acid labelled with a marker will identify viral nucleic acid.
- Polymerase chain reaction (PCR) can amplify small amounts of nucleic acid.

## HOST RESPONSE

### Antibody detection

- **Interpretation**:
  - **Immunoglobulin (Ig) M**: levels rise early and suggest recent or current infection.
  - **IgG**: must rise fourfold over a 2 week period to be diagnostic of a recent or current infection. Can also suggest previous infection.
- **ELISA**: see Chapter 1, Bacteria for further details.
- **Western blot**:
  - Electrophoresis is used to separate viral proteins in a gel solution.
  - These proteins are subsequently transferred (blotted) onto filter paper.
  - The sample serum is added to the paper; if viral antibodies are present, they will bind to the antigen.
  - This complex can be detected by adding a labelled antibody to human IgG and visualized in a similar manner to ELISA or immunofluorescence.

# 2.4 VIRUS IDENTIFICATION FLOWCHART (FIG. 2.3)

# 2.5 DNA VIRUSES

There are five key groups of DNA viruses:

1. *Herpesviridae*;
2. *Adenoviridae*;
3. *Parvoviridae*;
4. *Papovaviridae*;
5. *Hepadnaviridae.*

## HERPESVIRIDAE

All *Herpesviridae* are capable of latency periods and therefore persist lifelong.

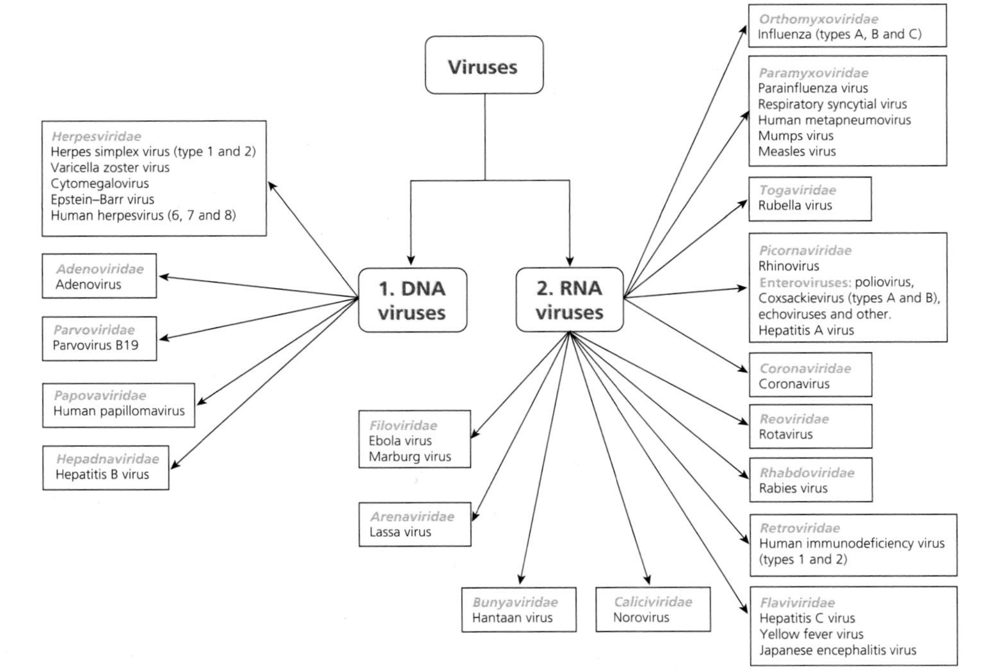


Fig. 2.3 Virus identification flowchart.

## Key examples

### *Herpes simplex virus*

- **Key features**:
  - There are two subtypes of herpes simplex virus (HSV): HSV-1 and HSV-2.
  - They are associated with different diseases, although they are not mutually exclusive (HSV-1 predominantly oral lesions and HSV-2 genital).
  - The virus can remain dormant in the sensory ganglia of the spinal cord.
  - The dormant virus can reactivate at a later stage.
  - Patients are infectious when they have active lesions.
  - Pregnant women with primary disease or current lesions are recommended to undergo elective lower segment caesarean section to prevent vertical transmission.
- **Transmission**:
  - **HSV-1**: saliva.
  - **HSV-2**: sexual intercourse.
- **Incubation period**: 2–12 days (for primary infection).
- **Diseases**:
  - **HSV-1**:
    - **Gingivostomatitis**: occurs with primary HSV infection; common in younger children; yellow vesicles in the mouth that become painful ulcers.
    - **Herpes labialis (cold sores)**: viral reactivation leads to vesicles that ulcerate and then crust, commonly on the lips.
    - Genital herpes, although usually HSV-2 (see Chapter 11, Genitourinary infections).
    - **Keratitis**: inflammation of the cornea with dendritic ulcers.
  - **HSV-2**:
    - genital herpes (see Chapter 11, Genitourinary infections);
    - herpes labialis (cold sores), although usually HSV-1;
    - neonatal infection.
  - **HSV-1 and HSV-2**:
    - Acute encephalitis (see Chapter 12, Nervous system infections).
    - Viral meningitis (see Chapter 12, Nervous system infections).
    - **Eczema herpeticum**: infection of eczema lesions.
    - **Herpetic whitlows**: herpetic lesions on the hands and fingers following manual contact with the virus.
    - **Systemic infection**: common among immunocompromised; can infect multiple organs.
- **Diagnosis**: isolation in cell culture, ELISA and immunofluorescence.
- **Anti-microbial**: aciclovir or famciclovir or valaciclovir.

*Varicella zoster virus*

- **Key features**:
  - Varicella zoster virus (VZV) can remain dormant in the sensory ganglia of the spinal cord and reactivate at a later stage.
  - Primary infection is more common in children but can also occur in adults and is usually more severe.
- **Transmission**: respiratory droplet spread.
- **Incubation period**: 13–21days.
- **Diseases**:
  - Chickenpox (varicella).
  - Shingles (zoster) (see Chapter 13, Skin infections).
  - Meningitis (see Chapter 12, Nervous system infections).
  - **Immunocompromised**: haemorrhagic lesions and pneumonitis.
- **Diagnosis**: majority of diagnosis based on clinical grounds or isolation in cell culture and immunofluorescence.
- **Anti-microbial**:
  - **Children**: calamine lotion or chlorphenamine.
  - **Adolescents/adults**: aciclovir.
  - **Exposed non-immune pregnant women**: varicella zoster immunoglobulin and aciclovir.

*Cytomegalovirus*

- **Key features**:
  - primary infection often asymptomatic;
  - lies dormant in the sensory ganglia after primary infection.
- **Transmission**: contact with infected secretions (e.g. saliva, urine and semen), transplacentally and through blood transfusions or organ transplants.
- **Incubation period**: 3–8 weeks.
- **Diseases**:
  - Congenital infection (cytomegalic inclusion disease).
  - **Immunocompetent**: mononucleosis-like syndrome with pharyngitis, lymphadenopathy and hepatitis.
  - **Immunocompromised**: encephalitis, pneumonitis, hepatitis and retinitis.
- **Diagnosis**: owl's eye inclusion bodies seen on tissue biopsy and PCR.
- **Anti-microbial**:
  - **Immunocompetent**: supportive, disease is self-limiting.
  - **Immunocompromised**: ganciclovir.

*Epstein–Barr virus*

- **Key features**: Epstein–Barr virus (EBV) infects B lymphocytes and epithelial cells in the oropharynx and nasopharynx.
- **Transmission**: contact with infected saliva (also called the kissing disease).

- **Incubation period**: 30–45 days.
- **Diseases**:
  - Infectious mononucleosis (glandular fever syndrome) (see Chapter 7, Respiratory infections).
  - Oral hairy leucoplakia.
  - **Associated pathology**:
    - Burkitt's lymphoma;
    - Hodgkin's lymphoma;
    - nasopharyngeal carcinoma.
- **Diagnosis**: lymphocytosis, atypical lymphocytes, positive monospot test (heterophil antibodies to EBV agglutinate horse blood) and IgM antibody to virus capsid antigen.
- **Anti-microbial**: none.

#### *Human herpesvirus*

- **Key features**: there are three key types of human herpesvirus (HHV): types 6, 7 and 8.
- **Transmission**: contact with infected saliva.
- **Diseases**:
  - **HHV-6 and HHV-7**: roseola infantum (exanthem subitum).
  - **HHV-8**: Kaposi's sarcoma.

## *ADENOVIRIDAE*

### Key example

#### *Adenovirus*

- **Key features**: there are 41 serotypes of adenovirus resulting in a broad range of pathology.
- **Transmission**: respiratory droplet spread and faecal–oral.
- **Incubation period**: 2–14 days.
- **Diseases**:
  - **Eye**: conjunctivitis.
  - **Gastrointestinal**: gastroenteritis, hepatitis and mesenteric adenitis.
  - **Respiratory**: common cold, pharyngitis, bronchitis, bronchiolitis and pneumonia (see Chapter 7, Respiratory infections).
- **Diagnosis**: isolation in cell culture from throat swab or faeces and immunofluorescence.

## *PARVOVIRIDAE*

### Key example

#### *Parvovirus B19*

- **Transmission**: respiratory droplet spread or direct contact with infected secretions.

- **Incubation period**: 18 days maximum.
- **Diseases**:
  - Erythema infectiosum (also known as slapped cheek disease and fifth disease) (see Chapter 15, Congenital, neonatal and childhood infections).
  - **Aplastic crisis**: affects individuals with sickle cell anaemia and thalassaemia.
- **Diagnosis**: ELISA testing for antibodies

## *PAPOVAVIRIDAE*

### Key example

#### *Human papillomaviruses*

- **Key features**: over 70 subtypes have been discovered.
- **Transmission**: direct contact with infected secretions (not blood).
- **Incubation period**: development of warts can occur from 1 to 20 months after exposure.
- **Diseases**:
  - Papilloma (common wart) (see Chapter 11, Genitourinary infections).
  - **Associated pathology**:
    - cervical cancer;
    - oral cancer.
- **Diagnosis**: koliocytosis (squamous cell dysplasia).
- **Anti-microbial**:
  - **Immunization (UK schedule)**: girls between 12 and 13 years old.

> **MICRO-facts**
>
> Human papillomavirus (HPV) serotypes **16** and **18** cause the majority of **cervical cancers**. The **vaccine** targets these serotypes (also types **6 and 11**).

## *HEPADNAVIRIDAE*

### Key example

#### *Hepatitis B virus*

- **Key features**:
  - Hepatitis B is the only DNA hepatitis virus, the others are all RNA viruses.
  - Three hepatitis B antigens are useful in assessing the status of the disease. They include: the surface antigen, the e antigen and the core antigen.
- **Transmission**: contact with infected blood products or sexual intercourse.

- **Incubation period**: 2–6 months.
- **Diseases**:
  - **Gastrointestinal**: infective hepatitis (acute and chronic) and hepatocellular carcinoma (see Chapter 8, Gastrointestinal infections).
- **Diagnosis**: detection of hepatitis B antigens in serum.
- **Anti-microbial**:
  - **Chronic hepatitis B**: peginterferon alfa-2a or interferon alfa or adefovir dipivoxil or lamivudine.
  - **Immunization**: offered to high-risk groups (e.g. healthcare professionals and intravenous drug users).

## 2.6 RNA VIRUSES

There are 10 key groups of RNA viruses:

1. *Orthomyxoviridae*;
2. *Paramyxoviridae*;
3. *Togaviridae*;
4. *Picornaviridae*;
5. *Coronaviridae*;
6. *Reoviridae*;
7. *Rhabdoviridae*;
8. *Retroviridae*;
9. *Flaviviridae*;
10. *Caliciviridae.*

### *ORTHOMYXOVIRIDAE*

#### Key example

*Influenza virus (types A, B and C)*

- **Key features**:
  - Common in winter months.
  - The influenza virus is subtyped by variations in the two glycoproteins (HA and neuraminidase (NA)) found in its lipid envelope.
  - Point mutations lead to changes in HA and NA and therefore undermine previous humoral immunity; this can result in an epidemic (also called antigenic drift).
  - Influenza virus type A is capable of a process called antigenic shift, in which new antigens are formed by genetic recombination. This can result in pandemics such as the Spanish flu (1918).
  - Swine flu (H1N1) and avian influenza (H5N1) are both caused by an influenza virus that has interacted with animal influenza viruses.

- **Transmission**: respiratory droplet spread or direct contact with infectious material.
- **Incubation period**: 1–5 days.
- **Diseases**:
  - **Respiratory**: influenza (see Chapter 7, Respiratory infections).
- **Diagnosis**: clinical diagnosis or viral isolation in tissue culture, immunofluorescence of nasal samples and complement fixation tests.
- **Anti-microbial**:
  - **Immunization**:
    - offered to people over 65 years old, healthcare professionals and those with chronic diseases (e.g. cystic fibrosis, renal disease and heart disease);
    - the vaccine protects against types A and B and is changed annually based on predictions of the strain likely to be most prevalent.
  - **NA inhibitors**:
    - **Examples**: oseltamivir (Tamiflu).
    - Decrease duration and severity of infection.

## PARAMYXOVIRIDAE

### Key examples

#### *Parainfluenza virus*

- **Transmission**: respiratory droplet spread.
- **Incubation period**: 2–6 days.
- **Diseases**:
  - **Respiratory**: laryngotracheobronchitis (croup), common cold, bronchiolitis and pneumonia (see Chapter 7, Respiratory infections).
  - **Diagnosis**: isolation in cell culture with haemadsorption or immunofluorescence.

#### *Respiratory syncytial virus*

- **Key features**:
  - Winter epidemics of RSV bronchiolitis are common in the UK.
  - Children with bronchopulmonary dysplasia and congenital heart disease are especially susceptible to RSV infection.
- **Transmission**: respiratory droplet spread.
- **Incubation period**: 2–6 days.
- **Diseases**:
  - **Respiratory**: bronchiolitis, laryngotracheobronchitis and common cold (see Chapter 7, Respiratory infections).
- **Diagnosis**: isolation in cell culture and immunofluorescence.

- **Anti-microbial**:
  - **Monoclonal antibody**: may be given to high-risk children.

> **MICRO-print**
>
> *HUMAN METAPNEUMOVIRUS*
>
> **Key features:** recently discovered virus that causes similar conditions to respiratory syncytial virus.
> **Transmission:** respiratory droplet spread.
> **Diseases:**
> **Respiratory:** bronchiolitis and common cold.

*Mumps virus*

- **Key features**: the mumps virus is highly contagious and can therefore spread rapidly through close communities.
- **Transmission**: respiratory droplet spread.
- **Incubation period**: 12–25 days.
- **Diseases**: mumps (see Chapter 15, Congenital, neonatal and childhood infections).
- **Diagnosis**: isolation in cell culture with haemadsorption.
- **Anti-microbial**:
  - **Immunization (UK schedule)**: 13 months, and 3 years and 4 months.

> **MICRO-facts**
>
> Mumps can cause bilateral orchitis and subsequent infertility.

*Measles virus*

- **Transmission**: respiratory droplet spread.
- **Incubation period**: 7–18 days.
- **Diseases**: measles (rubeola) (see Chapter 15, Congenital, neonatal and childhood infections).
- **Diagnosis**: ELISA testing for measles IgG and immunofluorescence to detect measles antigen.
- **Anti-microbial**:
  - **Immunization (UK schedule)**: 13 months, and 3 years and 4 months.

## TOGAVIRIDAE

### Key example

*Rubella virus*

- **Transmission**: respiratory droplet spread and transplacentally.
- **Incubation**: 16–18 days.

- **Diseases**:
  - Rubella (German measles) (see Chapter 15, Congenital, neonatal and childhood infections).
  - Congenital rubella syndrome.
- **Diagnosis**:
  - **Acute infection**: ELISA detection of IgM antibody.
  - **Immune status**: detection of IgG antibody by ELISA or latex agglutination test.
- **Anti-microbial**:
  - **Immunization (UK schedule)**: 13 months, and 3 years and 4 months.

## *PICORNAVIRIDAE*

### Key examples

#### *Rhinovirus*

- **Key features**:
  - principal cause of the common cold;
  - over 100 serotypes exist so the common cold remains common;
  - unable to withstand gastric acid, unlike other *Picornaviridae.*
- **Transmission**: respiratory droplet spread or direct contact with infectious material.
- **Incubation period**: 1–4 days.
- **Diagnosis**: clinical diagnosis. Rhinovirus can be grown in the laboratory but this technique is rarely used.
- **Diseases**:
  - **Respiratory**: common cold (see Chapter 7, Respiratory infections).

#### *Enteroviruses (including poliovirus, Coxsackievirus (A and B), echovirus and other enteroviruses)*

- **Key features**:
  - There are several forms of all the enteroviruses.
  - They replicate in the epithelial lining of respiratory and gastrointestinal tracts.
- **Transmission**: faecal–oral.
- **Incubation period**: 2–5 days.
- **Diseases**:
  - **Poliovirus**: poliomyelitis (see Chapter 12, Nervous system infections).
  - **Coxsackievirus (A and B)**:
    - Meningitis (see Chapter 12, Nervous system infections).
    - **Hand, foot and mouth disease**: caused by Coxsackievirus A16; vesicles develop on the palms, soles and tongue.
    - **Herpangia**: caused by Coxsackievirus A; painful vesicles develop on the palate and uvula.

- **Echovirus**:
  - myocarditis;
  - meningitis;
  - encephalitis;
  - acute non-specific febrile illness, commonly in younger children.
- **Other enteroviruses**:
  - ***Enterovirus* 70**: acute haemorrhagic conjunctivitis.
  - ***Enterovirus* 71**: hand, foot and mouth disease, meningitis, encephalitis and diarrhoea.

- **Anti-microbial**:
  - **Poliovirus immunization (UK schedule)**: 2, 3 and 4 months; 3 years and 4 months; and 13–18 years old.

#### *Hepatitis A virus*

- **Transmission**: faecal–oral.
- **Incubation period**: 2–6 weeks.
- **Diseases**:
  - **Gastrointestinal**: infective hepatitis (acute only) (see Chapter 8, Gastrointestinal infections).
- **Diagnosis**: detection of IgM antibody suggests acute infection.
- **Anti-microbial**:
  - **Immunization**: offered to high-risk groups (e.g. travellers).

## *CORONAVIRIDAE*

### Key example

#### *Coronavirus*

- **Transmission**: respiratory droplet spread.
- **Incubation period**: 2–5 days.
- **Diseases**: common cold (see Chapter 7, Respiratory infections).

## *REOVIRIDAE*

### Key example

#### *Rotavirus*

- **Key features**: able to survive stomach acid and replicate in small intestine mucosa.
- **Transmission**: faecal–oral.
- **Incubation period**: 1–2 days.
- **Diagnosis**: ELISA to demonstrate virus in stool sample.
- **Diseases**:
  - **Gastrointestinal**: gastroenteritis.

## *RHABDOVIRIDAE*

### Key example

*Rabies virus*

- **Key features**: without treatment, mortality associated with rabies is close to 100%.
- **Transmission**: bite from infected animal (e.g. dogs, cats and bats).
- **Incubation period**: 3–78 days.
- **Diseases**: rabies.
- **Diagnosis**: detection of Negri bodies (cytoplasmic inclusion bodies) in a stained tissue sample.
- **Anti-microbial**:
  - Rabies-specific immunoglobulin.
  - **Immunization**: a vaccine is available for high-risk groups (e.g. travellers).

## *RETROVIRIDAE*

### Key example

*Human immunodeficiency virus (types 1 and 2)*

- **Key features**:
  - HIV weakens the immune system by destroying T-helper (CD4) cells and can ultimately lead to acquired immune deficiency syndrome (AIDS).
  - HIV is a retrovirus; it makes use of the enzyme reverse transcriptase to convert its viral RNA into DNA for the purposes of cell replication.
  - Two serotypes exist: HIV-1 and HIV-2.
- **Transmission**: blood contact with infected bodily secretions (blood, semen and breast milk), e.g. needle sharing, sexual intercourse or perinatally.
- **Incubation period**: 2–4 weeks.
- **Diseases**: HIV and AIDS (see Chapter 10, Haematological infections and HIV).
- **Diagnosis**: detecting viral antibodies by ELISA (initially) and western blot (confirmatory).
- **Anti-microbial**: anti-retroviral drugs.

## *FLAVIVIRIDAE*

### Key example

*Hepatitis C virus*

- **Transmission**: contact with infected blood products or sexual intercourse.
- **Incubation period**: 2–26 weeks.

- **Diseases**:
  - **Gastrointestinal**: infective hepatitis (acute and chronic) and hepato-cellular carcinoma (see Chapter 8, Gastrointestinal infections).
- **Diagnosis**: detection of viral antibody by ELISA.
- **Anti-microbial**: ribavirin and peginterferon alfa.

**MICRO-print**

**YELLOW FEVER VIRUS**

**Key features:** restricted to tropical areas (e.g. Africa and south America).
**Transmission:** mosquito bite.
**Diseases:** yellow fever (jaundice, fever, headache, gastrointestinal haemorrhage and eventual multiorgan failure).
**Anti-microbial:** vaccination only.

**JAPANESE ENCEPHALITIS VIRUS**

**Transmission:** mosquito bite, primarily found in Asian rice fields.
**Diseases:** encephalitis.
**Anti-microbial:** vaccination only.

## *CALICIVIRIDAE*

### Key example

*Norovirus (also small round structured virus or Norwalk-like virus)*

- **Key features**:
  - causes outbreaks of gastroenteritis in winter;
  - norovirus is highly infectious so spreads rapidly through close communities (e.g. hospitals).
- **Transmission**: faecal–oral.
- **Incubation period**: 16–48 hours.
- **Diagnosis**: clinical.
- **Diseases**:
  - **Gastrointestinal**: winter vomiting (vomiting, diarrhoea and fever) (see Chapter 8, Gastrointestinal infections).

**MICRO-print**

***FILOVIRIDAE***

Key examples

**Ebola virus:**
**Transmission:** bodily fluids including blood.
**Diseases:** Ebola haemorrhagic fever.

*continued...*

*continued...*

**Marburg virus:**
**Transmission:** bodily fluids including blood.
**Diseases:** Marburg haemorrhagic fever.

***ARENAVIRIDAE***

Key example
**Lassa virus:**
**Transmission:** food and water contaminated with rodent urine.
**Diseases:** viral haemorrhagic fever.

***BUNYAVIRIDAE***

Key example
**Hantaan virus:**
**Transmission:** inhalation of aerosolized rodent's urine or faeces.
**Diseases:** Korean haemorrhagic fever.

# 3 Fungi

## 3.1 FUNGI CLASSIFICATION

Fungi are eukaryotic organisms that can be subdivided into three clinically relevant groups.

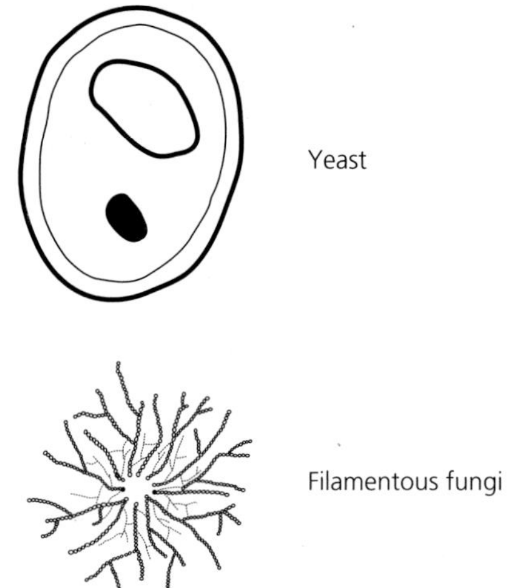


Fig. 3.1 Fungi shapes.

### YEASTS

- **Key examples**:
  - *Candida* spp. (also capable of producing pseudohyphae; therefore, often referred to as yeast like).
  - *Cryptococcus* spp.
- **Structure**: single round or oval cells.
- **Reproduction**: asexually through budding to produce blastospores (conidia).

### FILAMENTOUS FUNGI (MOULDS)

- **Key examples**:
  - *Aspergillus* spp.;
  - dermatophytes (also ringworm fungi – collective term for a range of fungi that cause superficial skin infections).
- **Structure**: grow by producing hyphae, a long filamentous cell that forms a network-like structure called a mycelium.
- **Reproduction**: asexually through budding to produce spores (conidia).

### ATYPICAL FUNGI

- **Key examples**:
  - *Pneumocystis* spp.;
  - *Histoplasma* spp.

## 3.2 DIAGNOSIS OF FUNGAL INFECTIONS

There are three main techniques used to diagnose fungal infections in the laboratory: **microscopy**, **culture** and **nucleic acid tests**.

### MICROSCOPY

- Patient samples are often treated with potassium hydroxide to destroy non-fungal material.
- Some samples may be stained with dyes before being viewed under a light microscope.
- Characteristic morphology can aid the diagnosis of fungal infection.

### CULTURE

- Sabouraud's agar is often used to culture samples as the low pH and added antibiotics inhibit the growth of bacteria.
- Fungi require an aerobic environment to grow.

### NUCLEIC ACID TESTS

- Polymerase chain reaction (PCR) is occasionally used to diagnose *Candida* spp. and *Aspergillus* spp.

## 3.3 YEASTS

### *CANDIDA* SPP.

#### Key example

##### Candida albicans

- **Location**: normal flora of oropharynx, vagina and gastrointestinal tract.

- **Transmission**: infections can occur when normal bacterial flora is disrupted (e.g. antibiotic use, immunosuppression and pregnancy) or when immunity is altered.
- **Diseases**:
  - **Skin**: cutaneous candidiasis, candidal paronychia and nappy rash.
  - **Oral**: oral candidiasis (commonly associated with inhaled corticosteroids).
  - **Genitals**: candidal vulvitis and vaginal candidiasis (thrush) (see Chapter 11, Genitourinary infections).
  - **Urinary tract**: urinary tract infection (colonizes catheters) (see Chapter 11, Genitourinary infections).
  - **Gastrointestinal**: candidal oesophagitis (especially in immunocompromised patients).
  - **Prostheses**: intravenous line infection.
  - **Systemic**: multiple organ dissemination, especially in immunocompromised states.
- **Diagnosis**: cream colonies, Gram positive, germ tubes at 37°C (hyphae arising from round yeast cell) and PCR diagnosis.
- **Anti-microbial**:
  - **Skin**:
    - **Cutaneous candidiasis**: clotrimazole (topical).
  - **Oral**:
    - **Oral candidiasis**: nystatin (mouthwash) or amphotericin (lozenges) or fluconazole (tablets).
  - **Genitals**:
    - **Candidal vulvitis**: clotrimazole (topical).
    - **Vaginal candidiasis**: clotrimazole (pessary or cream) or fluconazole or itraconazole.
  - **Invasive candidiasis**: fluconazole or voriconazole/capsofungin (fluconazole resistant).

## *CRYPTOCOCCUS* SPP.

### Key example

Cryptococcus neoformans

- **Location**: bird droppings.
- **Transmission**: inhalation of spores.
- **Diseases**:
  - **Cryptococcosis** (rare except for immunocompromised states):
    - **Pulmonary**: ranges from minor flu-like symptoms to pneumonia or respiratory distress syndrome.
    - **Neurological**: meningitis.

Microbiology

- **Diagnosis**: visible under the microscope after spinal fluid stained with India ink and serological tests on spinal fluid.
- **Anti-microbial**: amphotericin B and flucytosine and then fluconazole.

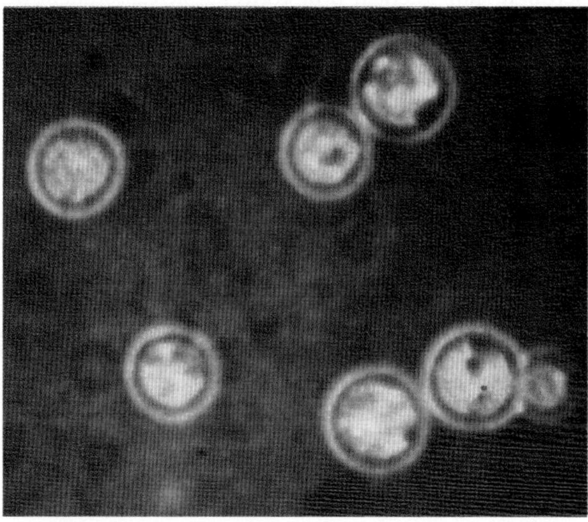

Fig. 3.2 *Cryptococcus neoformans*. Courtesy of the Academic Department of Infection & Immunity, University of Sheffield, UK.

## 3.4 FILAMENTOUS FUNGI

### *ASPERGILLUS* SPP.

#### Key example

Aspergillus fumigatus

- **Location**: airborne spores from soils, dusts and decaying vegetation.
- **Transmission**: inhalation of spores.
- **Diseases**:
  - **Allergic bronchopulmonary aspergillosis**: allergic reaction to *A. fumigatus* spores in asthmatic patients causes bronchospasm, fever and cough.
  - **Aspergilloma**: 'fungus ball' in pre-existing lung cavity (e.g. secondary to tuberculosis (TB)).
  - **Invasive aspergillosis**: patients almost always immunocompromised; systemic sepsis with *Aspergillus*.
- **Diagnosis**:
  - Microscopy: form branching hyphae (V-shaped), conidia extend from fungi.

  - Eosinophila.
  - Immunoglobulin (Ig) G precipitins test positive: may be positive in normal individuals, so correlate with clinical condition.
- **Anti-microbial**: amphotericin B or voriconazole/capsofungin (invasive aspergillosis).

### DERMATOPHYTES (RINGWORM FUNGI)

#### Key examples

Tricophyton *spp.,* Microsporum *spp. and* Epidermophyton *spp.*

- **Location**: humans, animals or soil.
- **Transmission**: direct skin contact with fungus.
- **Diseases**:
  - **Ringworm (tinea)**: classified according to infected site (e.g. tinea pedis is infection of the foot and colloquially referred to as athlete's foot).
- **Diagnosis**: microscopy with potassium hydroxide and culture on Sabouraud's agar.
- **Anti-microbial**: clotrimazole (topical) or terbinafine.

## 3.5 ATYPICAL FUNGI

### *PNEUMOCYSTIS* SPP.

#### Key example

Pneumocystis jiroveci (*previously* Pneumocystis carinii)

- The classification of *Pneumocystis* spp. has been a contentious subject since the 1980s. Originally believed to be protozoa, it has recently been reclassified as an atypical fungus.
- **Transmission**: respiratory droplet spread.
- **Diseases**:
  - **Respiratory**: *Pneumocystis carinii* pneumonia (only in immunocompromised states, especially human immunodeficiency virus) (see Chapter 10, Haematological infections and HIV).
- **Diagnosis**: bronchoalveolar lavage or transbronchial biopsies are stained with methenamine silver and viewed under a microscope and PCR detection.
- **Anti-microbial**: co-trimoxazole (trimethoprim and sulfamethoxazole).

### *HISTOPLASMA* SPP.

#### Key examples

Histoplasma capsulatum

- *H. capsulatum* is a diamorphic fungus. At body temperature it grows like a yeast and at 22–25°C (e.g. soil or artificial medium) it adopts a filamentous form.

- **Location**: soil.
- **Transmission**: inhalation of spores.
- **Diseases**:
    - **Histoplasmosis**: acutely infects the lungs, causing a pneumonia-like picture. Chronic pulmonary infection is similar to TB with cavitating lesions. Immunosuppressed individuals can develop disseminated disease affecting the lungs, liver, bone and brain.
- **Diagnosis**: microscopy or culture of sputum samples on Sabouraud's agar reveals *H. capsulatum* within macrophages.
- **Anti-microbial**: amphotericin B or itraconazole.

# 4 Protozoa

## 4.1 PROTOZOAL CLASSIFICATION

Protozoa are single-celled eukaryotes that can be classified according to their shape.

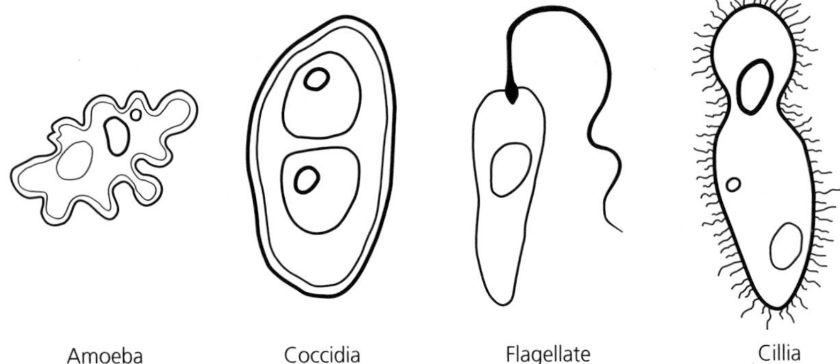


Fig. 4.1 Protozoal shapes.

### AMOEBA

- **Key examples**: *Entamoeba* spp.
- **Structure**: a cytoplasmic cellular membrane encloses cytoplasm, which contains a nucleus.
- **Movement**: pseudopods (literally, false feet) are formed in response to concentration gradients in the surrounding environment.
- **Life cycle** (two stages):
  - **Trophozoite**: the classical amoeba shape as shown in Fig. 4.1. The trophozoite is motile and able to feed.
  - **Cyst**: the infective form that is capable of surviving outside of the body.
- **Reproduction**: asexually through binary fission where one cell splits into two cells.

## COCCIDIA (SPOROZOA)

- **Key examples**: *Toxoplasma* spp., *Cryptosporidium* spp. and *Plasmodium* spp.
- **Life cycle**: coccidia have a multiple stage life cycle that occurs both within humans and in the environment:
  - **Oocyst**: this form is produced by gametogony and contains multiple sporozoites. Oocysts are able to withstand extreme environments and are commonly ingested in contaminated water. Once in the gastro-intestinal tract the sporozoites are released.
  - **Sporozoites**: this form invades the epithelial cells of the intestine.
  - **Trophozoite**: within the epithelial cell the sporozoites transform into a trophozoite that reproduces by schizogony to produce multiple merozoites.
  - **Merozoites**: multiple merozoites are released into the intestine where they fulfil two roles. First, some merozoites cause infection. Second, other merozoites develop into male and female gametocytes that eventually combine to form a zygote and later an oocyst. Some oocysts remain in the intestine and release further sporozoites.
- **Reproduction**: coccidia can reproduce either asexually (schizogony) or sexually (gametogony).

## FLAGELLATE

- **Key examples**: *Giardia* spp., *Trichomonas* spp., *Trypanosomiasis* spp. and *Leishmania* spp.
- **Movement**: the trophozoite form has flagella to propel it through its environment.
- **Life cycle**: *Giardia* spp. exist in two forms during their life cycle:
  - **Cyst**: the infective form that is capable of surviving outside of the body and is usually ingested in contaminated food or water.
  - **Trophozoite**: upon reaching the small intestine, two trophozoites are released from each cyst. Trophozoites attach to the intestinal mucosa by a sucking disk and replicate by binary fission. As the trophozoites reach the colon they form infective cysts that are passed in stools.

## CILIATE

- **Key examples**: *Balantidium* spp.
- **Structure**: characterized by multiple cilia attached to their outer surface.

# 4.2 AMOEBA

## ENTAMOEBA SPP.

### Key example

#### Entamoeba histolytica

- **Location**: cysts contaminate food and water.
- **Transmission**: faecal–oral.
- **Diseases**:
    - **Gastrointestinal**: amoebic dysentery and liver abscess (see Chapter 8, Gastrointestinal infections).
- **Diagnosis**: microscopy of stool sample reveals cysts or trophozoites.
- **Anti-microbial**:
    - **Gastrointestinal**:
        - **Amoebic dysentery**: metronidazole.
        - **Liver abscess**: metronidazole and tinidazole.

**MICRO-facts**

After malaria and schistosomiasis, *Entamoeba histolytica* is the leading cause of parasitic death.

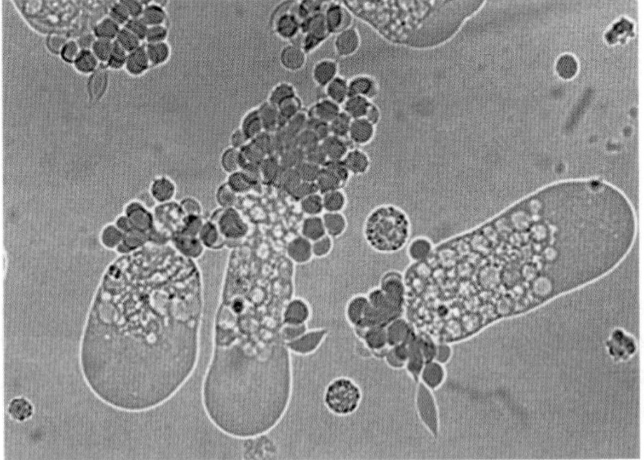

Fig. 4.2 *Entamoeba histolytica* trophozoites and red blood cells shown under microscopy. Courtesy of the Academic Department of Infection & Immunity, University of Sheffield, UK.

# 4.3 COCCIDIA (SPOROZOA)

## *TOXOPLASMA* SPP.

### Key example

#### Toxoplasma gondii

- **Location**: cat.
- **Transmission**: ingestion of cysts in cat faeces (e.g. food) or transplacentally (trophozoites).
- **Diseases**:
    - **Toxoplasmosis**:
        - **Immunocompetent**: asymptomatic or mononucleosis-type infection.
        - **Immunocompromised**: multisystem involvement including myocarditis, pneumonitis and encephalitis.
    - Congenital infection.
- **Diagnosis**: enzyme-linked immunosorbent assay (ELISA) testing for IgM and IgG antibodies.
- **Anti-microbial**: pyrimethamine and sulfadiazine.

## *CRYPTOSPORIDIUM* SPP.

### Key example

#### Cryptosporidium parvum

- **Location**: animal reservoir and contaminated water.
- **Transmission**: ingestion of water contaminated with cysts.
- **Diseases**: cryptosporidiosis (watery offensive stools with abdominal cramps).

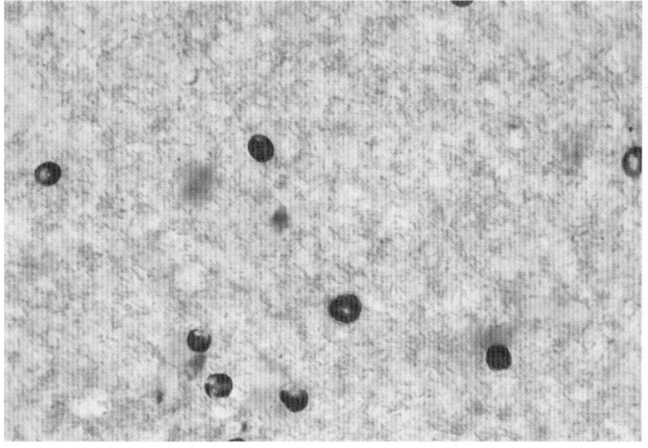

Fig. 4.3 *Cryptosporidium* spp. Courtesy of the Academic Department of Infection & Immunity, University of Sheffield, UK.

- **Diagnosis**: microscopy of a stool sample with an acid-fast stain shows oocytes.
- **Anti-microbial**:
  - **Immunocompetent**: self-limiting.
  - **Immunocompromised**: nitazoxanide.

### *PLASMODIUM* SPP.

#### Key examples

*Plasmodium falciparum, Plasmodium malariae, Plasmodium vivax* and *Plasmodium ovale*

- **Location**: female *Anopheles* mosquito or vertebrates.
- **Transmission**: inoculation by an infected female *Anopheles* mosquito.
- **Diseases**: malaria (see Chapter 10, Haematological infections and HIV).
- **Diagnosis**: thick and thin blood film.
- **Anti-microbial**: see Chapter 10, Haematological infections and HIV for more detail.

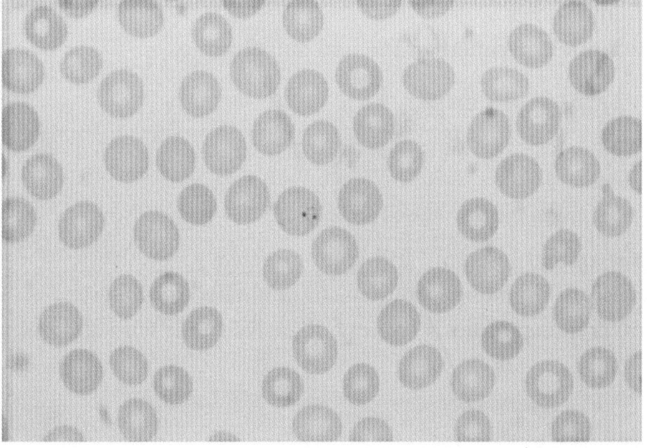

Fig. 4.4 *Plasmodium falciparum* on thin blood film (headphone-shaped microbe in central erythrocyte). Courtesy of the Academic Department of Infection & Immunity, University of Sheffield, UK.

## 4.4 FLAGELLATES

### *GIARDIA* SPP.

#### Key example

*Giardia lamblia*

- **Location**: contaminated water and animal reservoirs.
- **Transmission**: ingestion of contaminated water.
- **Diseases**: giardiasis (greasy diarrhoea, fatigue and bloating).

- **Diagnosis**: microscopy of stool sample shows trophozoites or cysts.
- **Anti-microbial**: metronidazole or tinidazole.

**MICRO-facts**

Chlorination of water does not kill *Giardia* spp.

## *TRICHOMONAS* SPP.

### Key example

Trichomonas vaginalis

- **Location**: human host.
- **Transmission**: sexual intercourse.
- **Diseases**: trichomoniasis (see Chapter 11, Genitourinary infections).
- **Diagnosis**: dark ground microscopy of genital secretion.
- **Anti-microbial**: metronidazole or tinidazole.

**MICRO-facts**

Trichomoniasis often causes a haemorrhagic cervix (known as a strawberry cervix).

**MICRO-print**

***TRYPANOSOMA*** spp.

Key examples

***Trypanosoma brucei***:
**Location:** tsetse fly, humans and animals.
**Transmission:** inoculation by an infected tsetse fly.
**Diseases:** African trypanosomiasis (sleeping sickness).
**Anti-microbial:** pentamidine isethionate or suramin or eflornithine.

***Trypanosoma cruzi***:
**Location:** domestic and wild animal reservoir and humans.
**Transmission:** inoculation by house-dwelling reduviid bugs.
**Diseases:** American trypanosomiasis (Chagas' disease).
**Anti-microbial:** benznidazole.

***LEISHMANIA*** SPP.
Key examples
***Leishmania donovani***:
**Transmission:** inoculation by female *Phlebotomus* sandfly.

*continued...*

*continued...*

**Diseases:** visceral leishmaniasis (kala-azar).
**Anti-microbial:** sodium stibogluconate or pentamidine isethionate.

***Leishmania tropica:***
**Transmission:** inoculation by female *Phlebotomus* sandfly.
**Diseases:** cutaneous leishmaniasis.
**Anti-microbial:** sodium stibogluconate.

***Leishmania braziliensis:***
**Transmission:** inoculation by female *Phlebotomus* sandfly.
**Diseases:** mucocutaneous leishmaniasis.
**Anti-microbial:** sodium stibogluconate or amphotericin B.

# 5 Helminths

## 5.1 HELMINTH CLASSIFICATION

There are three clinically relevant groups of helminths:
1. trematodes (flukes);
2. nematodes (roundworms);
3. cestodes (tapeworms).

## 5.2 TREMATODES (FLUKES)

### *SCHISTOSOMA* SPP.

#### Key examples

Schistosoma mansoni, Schistosoma haematobium *and* Schistosoma japonicum

- **Transmission**: infective cercariae penetrate skin.
- **Life cycle**:
  - cercariae penetrate skin;
  - migrate to bladder (*S. haematobium*) or intestine (*S. mansoni* and *S. japonicum*) via the bloodstream;
  - develop into male and female worms at these sites;
  - female form produces ova that are passed in urine or stools;
  - in fresh water, the ova hatch, releasing larvae that infect aquatic snails;
  - the larvae multiply within tropical aquatic snails to form infective cercariae.
- **Diseases**:
  - **Schistosomiasis**:
    - **All species**: dermatitis at the site of larvae penetration.
    - ***S. mansoni***: diarrhoea, rectal polyps, gastrointestinal fibrosis, hepatitis, portal hypertension and splenomegaly.
    - ***S. haematobium* (bilharzia)**: painless haematuria, increased urine frequency, obstructive uropathy results in hydronephrosis and renal failure. Chronic urinary schistosomiasis is associated with squamous cell carcinoma of the bladder.
    - ***S. japonicum***: similar symptoms to *S. mansoni* but more severe.

- **Diagnosis**: ova visible in stool or urine sample with microscopy and eosinophilia.
- **Anti-microbial**: praziquantel.

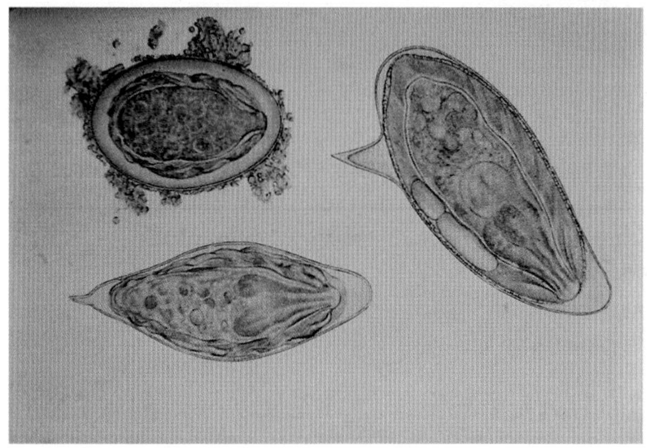

Fig. 5.1 *Schistosoma* spp. ova viewed under microscopy. Courtesy of the Academic Department of Infection & Immunity, University of Sheffield, UK.

## 5.3 NEMATODES (ROUNDWORMS)

### *ASCARIS* SPP.

#### Key example

Ascaris lumbricoides

- **Transmission**: ingestion of eggs in contaminated water, food or soil.
- **Life cycle**:
    - larvae hatch from ingested eggs in the intestinal mucosa;
    - migrate to lungs via the bloodstream;
    - expectorated and swallowed into stomach;
    - mature into adult worms in the gut and produce eggs that are released in faeces.
- **Clinical features**:
    - **Ascariasis**:
        - **Few worms**: asymptomatic.
        - **Greater parasitic load**: vomiting and abdominal discomfort.
        - **Complications**: pneumonitis, intestinal obstruction, malnutrition and hepatic abscess.
- **Diagnosis**: ova visible in stool sample with microscopy and eosinophilia.
- **Anti-microbial**: mebendazole or piperazine.

## *ENTEROBIUS* SPP.

### Key example

Enterobius vermicularis (*threadworm and pinworm*)

- **Transmission**: ingestion or inhalation of eggs present in environment.
- **Life cycle**:
  - larvae hatch from ingested eggs in the intestine and grow to adult form;
  - female worm lays eggs in peri-anal area that causes irritation and pruritus;
  - eggs become lodged under fingernails during scratching and are subsequently ingested.
- **Diseases**:
  - **Enterobiasis**: asymptomatic or pruritus ani.
- **Diagnosis**: ova found in the peri-anal region can be collected with the Scotch-tape technique or worms may be directly visible.
- **Anti-microbial**: mebendazole or piperazine.

> **MICRO-facts**
>
> **Threadworm** is the most common **helminth** in the UK.

## *TRICHURIS* SPP.

### Key example

Trichuris trichuria (*whipworm*)

- **Transmission**: ingestion of eggs in contaminated water, food or soil.
- **Life cycle**:
  - larvae hatch from ingested eggs in the small intestine and mature in the large intestine;
  - female worm produces eggs that are excreted into soil where they mature.
- **Diseases**:
  - **Trichuriasis**: asymptomatic or dysentery and anal prolapse.
- **Diagnosis**: ova visible in stool.
- **Anti-microbial**: oxantel pamoate.

## HOOKWORM

### Key examples

Ancylostoma duodenale *and* Necator americanus

- **Transmission**: infective larvae penetrate skin, especially feet.

- **Life cycle**:
  - larvae enter body through skin and migrate to lungs via bloodstream;
  - expectorated and swallowed into stomach;
  - mature into adult worms in the small intestine while taking blood meals;
  - eggs are passed in the stool.
- **Diseases**:
  - **Hookworm (ancylostomiasis and necatoriasis)**: irritation at entry site, abdominal pain, diarrhoea and iron-deficiency anaemia.
- **Diagnosis**: ova visible in stool with microscopy and eosinophilia.
- **Anti-microbial**: mebendazole or albendazole.

> **MICRO-facts**
>
> **Hookworm** is the most common cause of **iron-deficiency anaemia** in the **tropics**.

## *STRONGYLOIDES* SPP.

### Key example

#### Strongyloides stercoralis

- **Transmission**: infective larvae penetrate skin.
- **Life cycle**:
  - **External phase**:
    - Rhabditiform larvae are passed in the stool and develop into adult worms (male and female) or infective filariform larvae.
    - Adult worms produce eggs that become rhabditiform larvae and the cycle continues.
  - **Infective phase**:
    - Infective filariform larvae penetrate the skin and migrate to the lungs via the bloodstream.
    - Bronchial secretions containing the larvae are swallowed.
    - The female adult worm develops in the small intestine and produces rhabditiform larvae.
    - The larvae are passed in the stool (external phase continues) or develop into infective filariform larvae and autoinfect the host via the intestinal mucosa (internal) or peri-anal skin (external).
    - Autoinfective larvae can repeat the infective phase cycle or disseminate to distant organs.

- **Diseases**:
  - **Strongyloidiasis**:
    - Irritation and itch at entry site.
    - **Autoinfection**: serpiginous migratory urticarial rash on the buttocks and lower abdomen (pathognomonic).
    - **Gastrointestinal**: diarrhoea, malabsorption and perforation.
    - **Hyperinfestation syndrome**: mass bowel wall penetration in immunosuppressed patients causes severe infection and disseminated disease.
- **Diagnosis**: larvae visible in stool and eosinophilia.
- **Anti-microbial**: ivermectin or albendazole.

## FILARIASIS

### Key examples

*Wuchereria bancrofti* and *Brugia malayi* (lymphatic filariasis)

- **Transmission**: inoculation by infected mosquitoes.
- **Life cycle**:
  - immature larvae migrate to lymphatics and mature to adult form;
  - microfilariae are produced by fertilization and enter the bloodstream;
  - mosquitoes are reinfected when they take a blood meal.
- **Diseases**:
  - **Acute infection**: fever, malaise and lymphadenitis.
  - **Elephantitis**: severe peripheral oedema owing to blocked lymphatics and limb fibrosis.
- **Diagnosis**: clinical diagnosis, serological tests and eosinophilia.
- **Anti-microbial**: albendazole and diethylcarbamazine.

**MICRO-print**

***ONCHOCERCA VOLVULUS* (RIVER BLINDNESS)**

**Transmission:** inoculation by the black fly (breed near rivers).
**Life cycle:** microfilariae spread to distant skin sites and cause localized host response.
**Diseases:**
**Skin:** atrophy, lichenification and poor healing.
**Eye:** blindness.
**Diagnosis:** microfilaria visible in eye or skin shavings and eosinophilia.
**Anti-microbial:** ivermectin.

***LOA LOA***

**Transmission:** inoculation by infected *Chrysops* fly (mango fly).
**Life cycle:** larvae mature in subcutaneous tissue and produce microfilariae.

*continued...*

*continued...*

**Diseases:** loiasis (painful Calabar limb swellings and conjunctival infiltration).
**Diagnosis:** microfilariae visible in blood and eosinophilia.
**Anti-microbial:** diethylcarbamazine.

*TOXOCARA* **SPP.**

Key examples
***Toxocara cani*** and ***Toxocara cati***:
**Transmission:** ingestion of eggs.
**Life cycle:**
*Toxocara* spp. typically infect cats (*T. cati*) and dogs (*T. cani*).
Eggs are passed in faeces and can be ingested by humans.
Larvae penetrate the intestinal mucosa, pass to distant sites and form granulomas.
**Diseases:**
**Toxocariasis (visceral larva migrans):** bronchospasm, choroidoretinitis, hepatosplenomegaly and cardiac/neurological involvement (can be fatal).
**Diagnosis:** ELISA.
**Anti-microbial:** mebendazole.

## 5.4 CESTODES (TAPEWORMS)

**MICRO-facts**

All **tapeworms** are **hermaphrodites**.

### *TAENIA* SPP.

#### Key example

Taenia solium (*pork tapeworm*)

- **Location**: infected pigs or food and water contaminated with cysts.
- **Transmission**:
  - **Taeniasis**: ingestion of raw or undercooked pork containing cysticerci (larvae).
  - **Cysticercosis**: ingestion of food or water contaminated with eggs.
- **Life cycle**:
  - **Taeniasis:**
    - cysticerci are ingested from contaminated pork;
    - larvae mature into the adult form in the small intestine;

  - gravid terminal segments (proglottids) form the body of *T. solium* and contain multiple eggs. Sections are released and excreted in faeces;
  - pigs eat eggs and cysticerci form in the muscles (pork meat).
- **Cysticercosis**:
  - *T. solium* eggs are ingested and hatch into larvae in the intestine;
  - the larvae enter the bloodstream and travel to distant organs where an inflammatory response causes calcification.

- **Diseases**:
  - **Taeniasis (pork tapeworm)**: abdominal discomfort and diarrhoea.
  - **Cysticercosis**:
    - **Subcutaneous**: generally asymptomatic.
    - **Eye**: blindness.
    - **Neurocysticercosis**: hydrocephalus and epilepsy.
    - **Skeletal muscle**: majority asymptomatic.
- **Diagnosis**: gravid proglottids visible in a stool sample.
- **Treatment**:
  - **Taeniasis**: praziquantel or niclosamide.
  - **Cysticercosis**: praziquantel or albendazole.

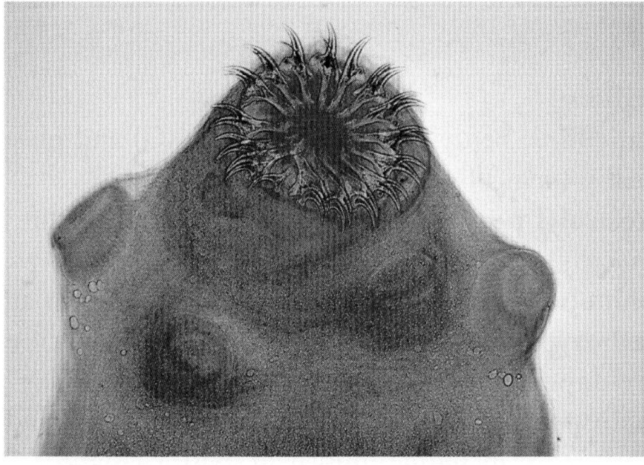

Fig. 5.2 *Taenia solium* scolex viewed under microscopy. Courtesy of the Academic Department of Infection & Immunity, University of Sheffield, UK.

# 6 Antibiotics

## 6.1 ANTIBIOTIC PHARMACODYNAMICS

Broadly, there are three key mechanisms by which antibiotics exert their anti-microbial effect.

### CELL WALL SYNTHESIS INHIBITORS

The bacterial cell wall is a natural target for anti-microbial treatment as its presence differentiates microbial cells from human cells and therefore diminishes potential toxic effects.

#### Key examples

*β-Lactams*

- **Examples**:
  - **Penicillins**:
    - **Penicillins**: benzylpenicillin (penicillin G) and phenoxymethylpenicillin (penicillin V).
    - **Isoxazolyl penicillins**: flucloxacillin and meticillin (not used clinically).
    - **Aminopenicillins**: ampicillin, amoxicillin and co-amoxiclav.
    - **Carboxypenicillin**: ticarcillin (with clavulanic acid).
    - **Ureidopenicillin**: piperacillin (with tazobactam).
  - **Cephalosporins**: including cephalexin, cefuroxime and ceftazidime.
  - **Carbapenems**: including imipenem (with cilastatin), ertapenem and meropenem.
- **Action**: these agents contain a β-lactam ring, which binds to penicillin-binding proteins (PBPs). PBPs are bacterial membrane proteins responsible for the final stages of cell wall creation, and their inhibition leads to a build-up of immature cell wall sections that eventually triggers cell autolysis.
- **Co-amoxiclav (Augmentin)**: amoxicillin combined with clavulanic acid, a β-lactamase inhibitor. It contains a β-lactam ring to bind with bacterial β-lactamase enzymes and prevent destruction of the amoxicillin molecule.

- **Piperacillin with tazobactam (Tazocin)**: tazobactam is a β-lactamase inhibitor that extends the spectrum of activity of piperacillin.
- **Imipenem with cilastatin**: cilastatin is an enzyme inhibitor that prevents rapid renal metabolism of imipenem and therefore increases serum concentrations.
- **Other**:
  - Cephalosporins and carbapenems are more resistant to β-lactamases than penicillins.
  - Piperacillin and ticarcillin are broad-spectrum penicillins that are particularly active against *Pseudomonas* spp. and anaerobes. They are reserved for severe infections.
  - Penicillin allergy also includes allergy to flucloxacillin, amoxicillin and ampicillin; 5% of patients will also be allergic to cephalosporins.

**MICRO-print**

**β-LACTAM GROUP**

The β-lactam group is subdivided according to the different rings and side chains attached to the β-lactam ring.

### *Glycopeptides*

- **Examples**: vancomycin and teicoplanin.
- **Action**: glycopeptides bind to the emerging cell wall structure, preventing further growth.
- **Other**:
  - Vancomycin and teicoplanin are active only against Gram-positive bacteria as their large size impairs their ability to penetrate Gram-negative cells.
  - Glycopeptides have poor oral availability so are given intravenously.
  - However, vancomycin is given orally in pseudomembranous colitis as it acts locally on the gastrointestinal tract.
  - They are poorly absorbed into the central nervous system.

**MICRO-facts**

**Vancomycin** can be **nephro**- and **ototoxic** and cause **red man syndrome** if given as a **bolus**.

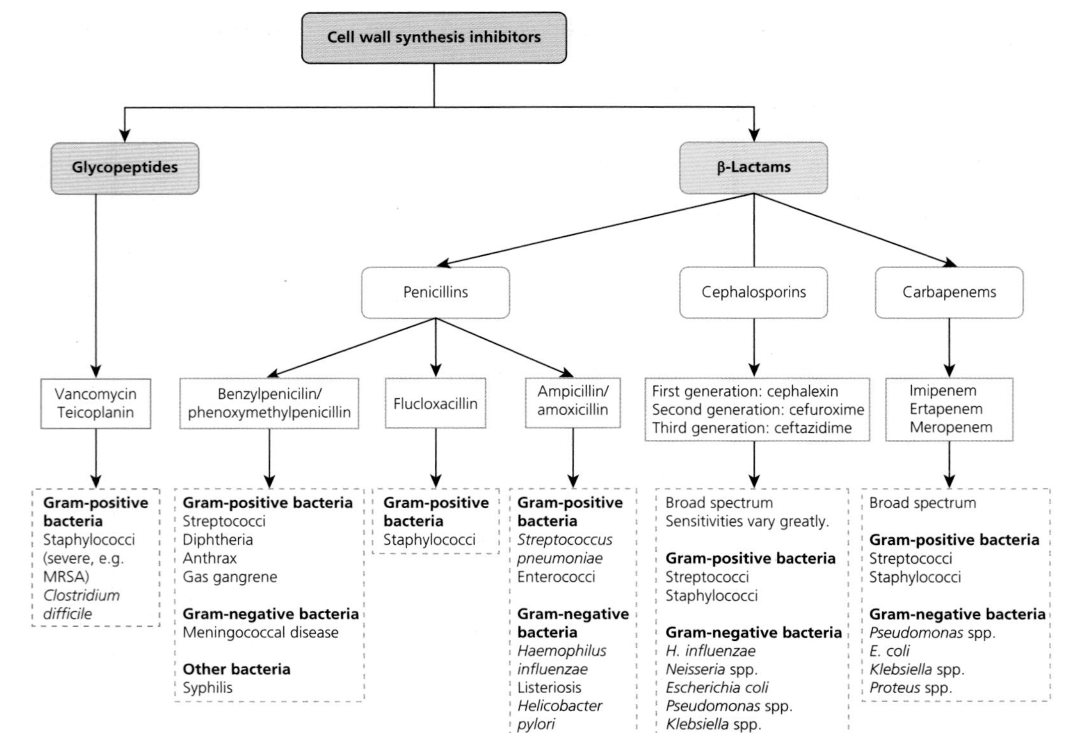


Fig. 6.1 Antibiotic mode of action and sensitivities: cell wall synthesis inhibitors. MRSA, meticillin-resistant *Staphylococcus aureus*.

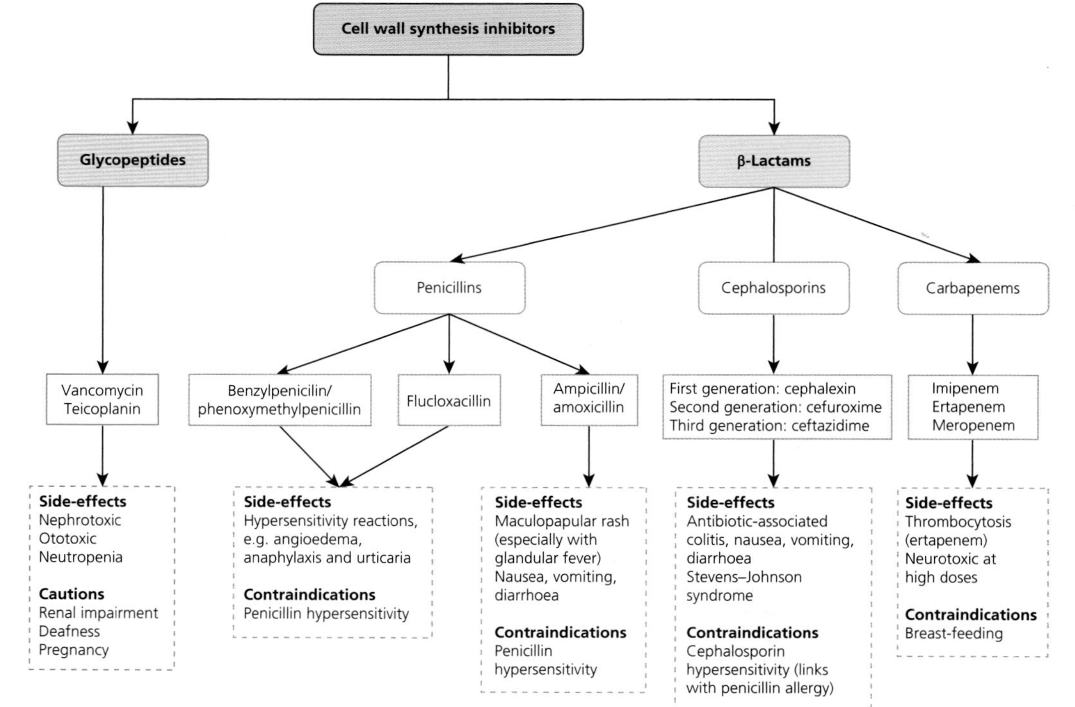


Fig. 6.2 Antibiotic side-effects and contraindications: cell wall synthesis inhibitors.

## NUCLEIC ACID SYNTHESIS INHIBITORS

### Key examples

#### *Sulfonamides*

- **Examples**: sulfadiazine.
- **Action**: sulfonamides are competitive receptor antagonists for the active site of the enzyme dihydropteroate synthetase. This enzyme is part of the pathway that produces tetrahydrofolic acid, a precursor of purines and pyrimidines, which are an integral part of nucleic acids (Fig. 6.3).
- **Other**: rarely used because of widespread resistance.

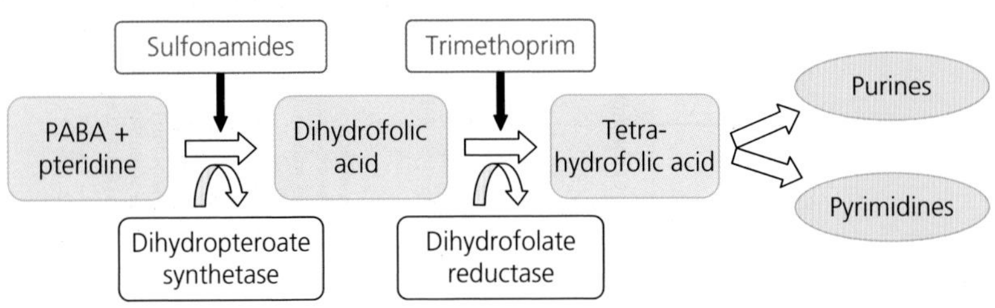


Fig. 6.3 Purine and pyrimidines synthesis pathway. PABA, *para*-aminobenzoic acid.

#### *Trimethoprim*

- **Action**: trimethoprim also disturbs the synthesis of purines and pyrimidines by inhibiting the enzyme dihydrofolate reductase (Fig. 6.3).
- **Co-trimoxazole**: a combination of sulfamethoxazole and trimethoprim used to treat *Pneumocystis jiroveci* (previously *Pneumocystis carinii*) pneumonia.

#### *Quinolones*

- **Examples**: ciprofloxacin, ofloxacin and levofloxacin.
- **Action**: interfere with two bacterial enzymes (deoxyribonucleic acid (DNA) gyrase and topoisomerases) that maintain the efficiency of DNA replication; therefore, causing the production of poor quality DNA strands.
- **Other**: the only true quinolones are the 'first-generation' drugs, such as nalidixic acid. All those that followed have been fluorinated (fluoroquinolones) to improve anti-bacterial activity.

#### *Rifamycins*

- **Example**: rifampicin.
- **Action**: rifampicin binds to ribonucleic acid (RNA) polymerase, therefore preventing mRNA synthesis.

- **Other**: it is given orally and is primarily used in the treatment of tuberculosis.

> **MICRO-facts**
>
> **Rifampicin** causes **orange-red** discolouration of **secretions** such as **saliva** and **urine**.

*Nitroimidazoles*

- **Example**: metronidazole.
- **Action**: these compounds enter the microbe and are then metabolized to an active form that breaks the cell's DNA.
- **Other**:
  - metronidazole is effective against anaerobic bacteria and parasites;
  - should not be mixed with alcohol as it interferes with alcohol metabolism, which results in a build-up of acetaldehyde, causing nausea, vomiting and flushing.

## PROTEIN SYNTHESIS INHIBITORS

This class of antibiotics is able to capitalize on slight differences between protein synthesis in bacterial and human cells to minimize damage to human cells.

### Key examples

*Chloramphenicol*

- **Action**: chloramphenicol binds to bacterial ribosome and interferes with the formation of peptide bonds in the expanding peptide chain.
- **Other**: chloramphenicol contains a nitrobenzene nucleus.

> **MICRO-print**
>
> **CHLORAMPHENICOL**
>
> It is the nitrobenzene nucleus that causes many of chloramphenicol's side-effects.

*Macrolides*

- **Examples**: erythromycin, azithromycin and clarithromycin.
- **Action**: binds to ribosomal RNA and prevents translocation.
- **Other**:
  - Macrolides contain a macrocyclic ring.

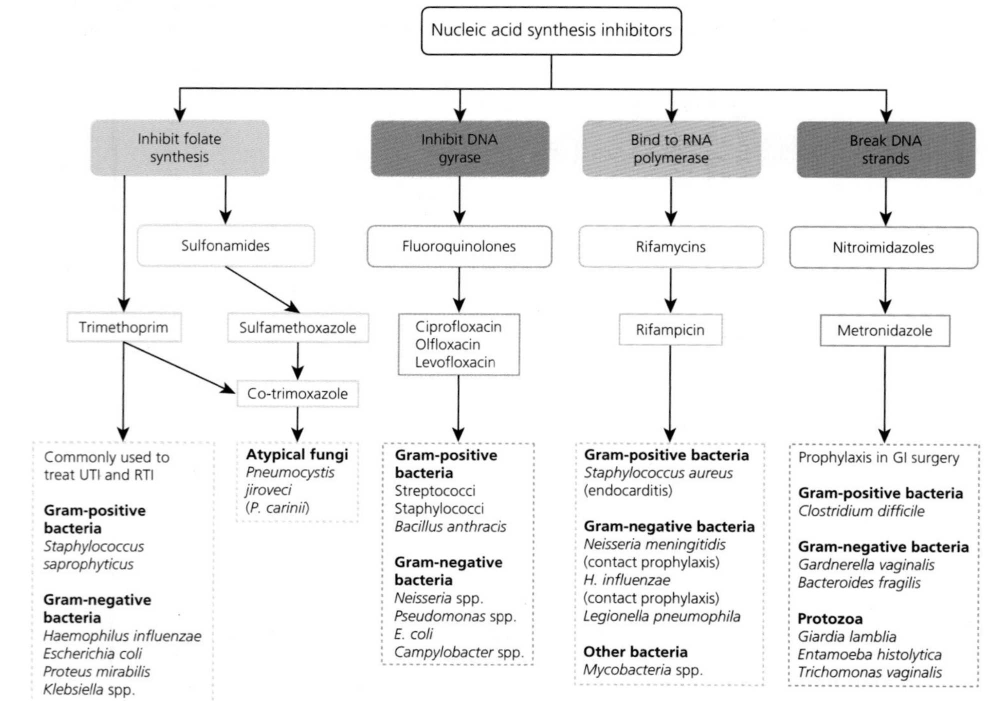


Fig. 6.4 Antibiotic mode of action and sensitivities: nucleic acid synthesis inhibitors. GI, gastrointestinal; RTI, respiratory tract infection; UTI, urinary tract infection.

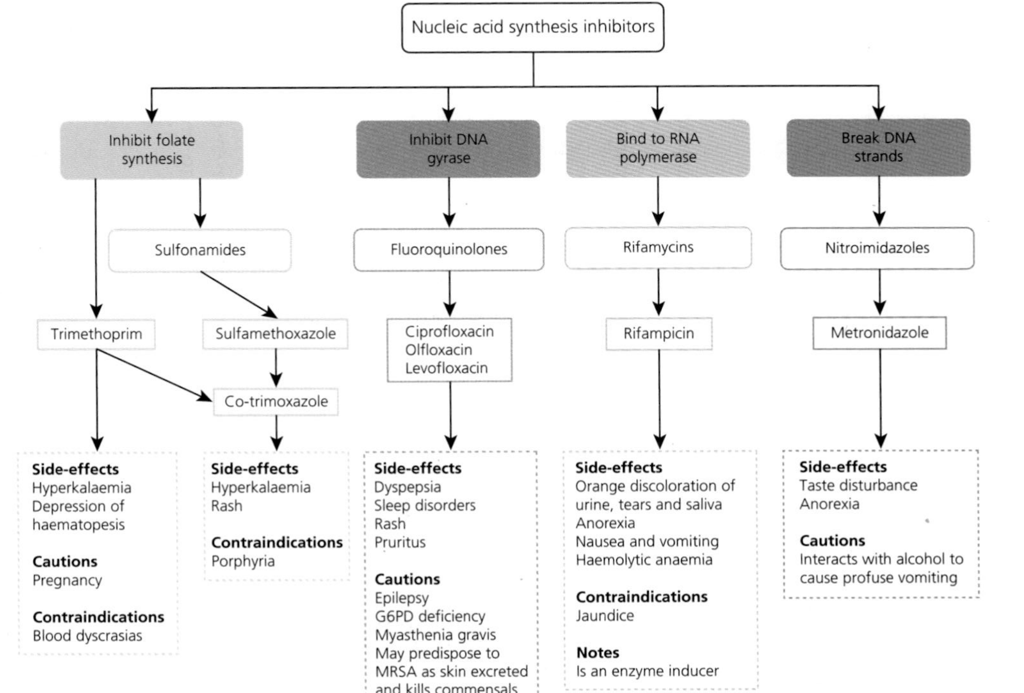


Fig. 6.5 Antibiotic side-effects and contraindications: nucleic acid synthesis inhibitors. G6PD, glucose-6-phosphate dehydrogenase; MRSA, meticillin-resistant *Staphylococcus aureus*.

- Azithromycin and clarithromycin can be given less frequently and are therefore useful when compliance may be an issue, such as treatment of chlamydia.
- Macrolides are poorly absorbed into the central nervous system.

> **MICRO-facts**
>
> **Erythromycin** has a **similar spectrum of activity** to **penicillins** so is a useful alternative in **penicillin allergy**.

*Lincosamides*

- **Examples**: clindamycin.
- **Action**: similar to macrolides.
- **Other**:
  - A common cause of *Clostridium difficile* pseudomembranous colitis.
  - Good bone penetration and *Staphylococcus* spp. activity make clindamycin a prime choice for osteomyelitis.

*Aminoglycosides*

- **Examples**: gentamicin and streptomycin.
- **Action**: normally protein synthesis is initiated by transfer RNA (tRNA) binding to ribosomes and forming initiation complexes. Aminoglycosides bind to these bacterial ribosomes (which are smaller than eukaryotic equivalents) and therefore prevent the initiation of protein production.
- **Other**:
  - Aminoglycosides should be given through an intravenous infusion as they are not absorbed orally.
  - Gentamicin levels should be monitored regularly to ensure that drug levels are within the narrow therapeutic range and to prevent ototoxicity and nephrotoxicity.

*Tetracyclines*

- **Examples**: tetracycline, doxycycline and oxytetracycline.
- **Action**: tetracyclines behave in a similar manner to aminoglycosides; they also prevent the attachment of a tRNA to the bacterial ribosome.
- **Other**: administration is usually oral.

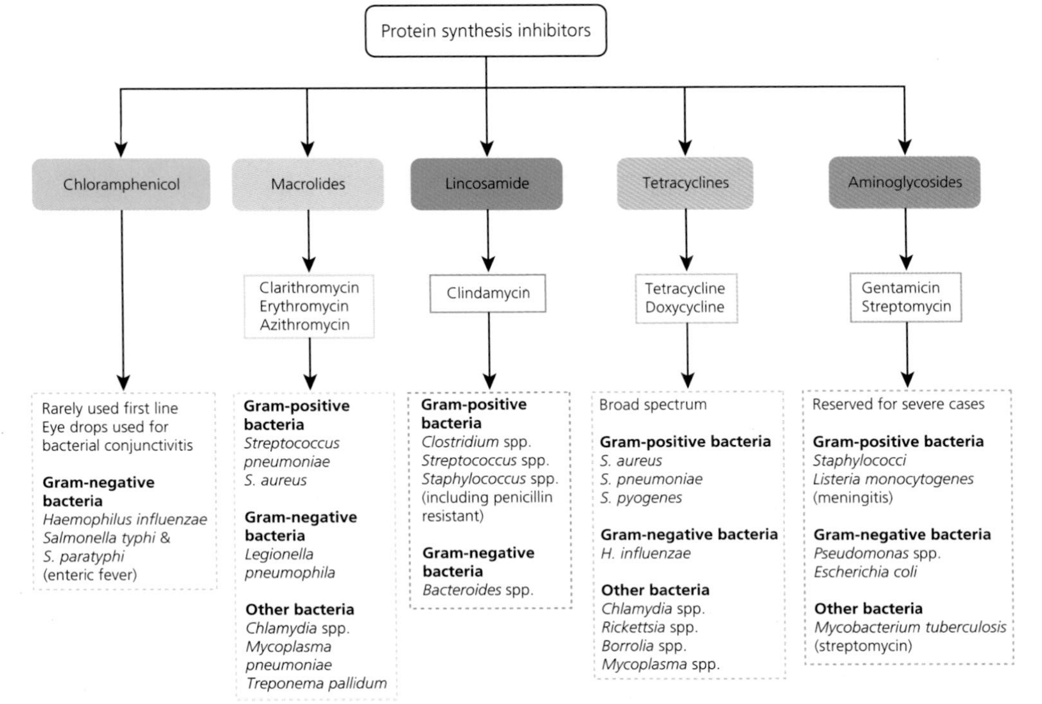


Fig. 6.6 Antibiotic mode of action and sensitivities: protein synthesis inhibitors.

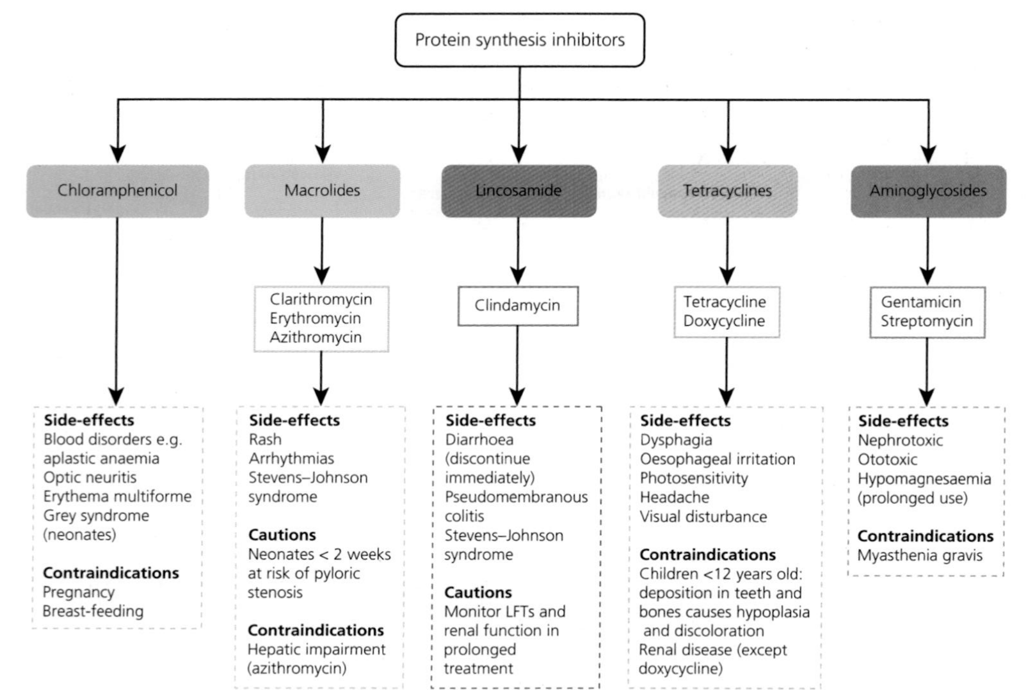


Fig. 6.7 Antibiotic side-effects and contraindications: protein synthesis inhibitors. LFTs, liver function tests.

## 6.2 ANTIBIOTIC RESISTANCE

Antibiotic resistance is a growing problem that poses a serious threat to the treatment of many severe illnesses.

### THE DEVELOPMENT OF ANTIBIOTIC RESISTANCE

There are three key genetic mechanisms by which antibiotic resistance develops.

#### Plasmid-mediated resistance

- This occurs when plasmids (portions of genetic information separate from the organism's chromosomal DNA) coding for antibiotic resistance mutations are passed between bacteria.
- Plasmids can be transferred between bacteria by pili.

#### Single or multiple chromosomal mutations

- Chromosomal mutations (often by chance) can give rise to resistance to antibiotics.

#### Jumping genes or transposons

- Jumping genes are so named as they can be transposed to different locations in the genome.
- These genes are able to integrate themselves into chromosomal DNA or onto plasmids and are then spread among a species, or even cross species.

### THE MECHANISMS OF ANTIBIOTIC RESISTANCE

On a molecular level, there are three key mechanisms by which microbes can impair the function of antibiotics and therefore demonstrate resistance:

1. **Changing the target site**: the specific area that an antibiotic will target may be altered, often meaning that the antibiotic is less likely to interact with it.
2. **Limiting access to the target site**: access to the specific site where the antibiotic exerts its influence may be limited. This can occur either by allowing less antibiotic to pass through the cell wall or by causing more to leave once it is inside.
3. **Antibiotic inactivation**: the organism may start to produce new enzymes that prevent the antibiotic from working (e.g. β-lactamases inactivate the β-lactam ring).

### THE β-LACTAM EXAMPLE

The β-lactams provide an important example of antibiotic resistance. Although this class of drugs are widely used in clinical practice, resistance by all three mechanisms described above has developed.

- **Changing the target site**: β-lactams normally target penicillin-binding proteins (PBPs), but methicillin-resistant *Staphylococcus aureus* is capable of producing alternative PBP that β-lactams are less able to bind with. This allows cell wall production to continue.
- **Limiting access to the target site**: in Gram-negative bacteria the PBPs are located on the inner membrane; therefore, β-lactams have to pass through the outer membrane to reach their target. Normally, this occurs by diffusion through porins (protein channels) but mutations allow some bacteria to block this process.
- **Antibiotic inactivation**: some bacteria are able to produce β-lactamases; these are enzymes that lead to the destruction of the β-lactam ring.

### MICRO-facts

There are multiple **β-lactamases**. Some work only on **specific β-lactams** whereas **extended-spectrum β-lactamases** imply resistance against **most β-lactams**; accordingly, these microbes are clinically challenging to treat.

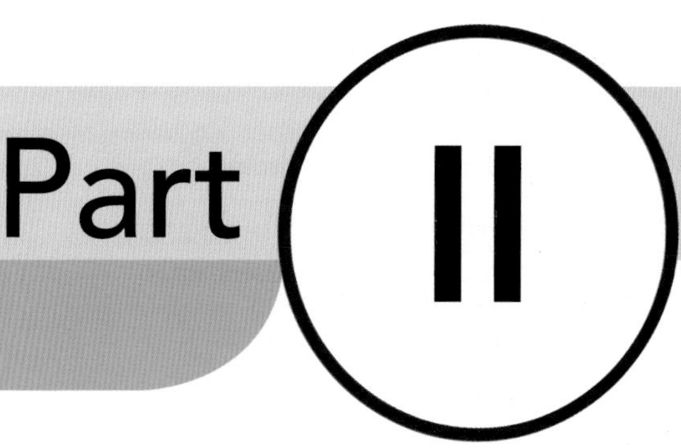


# Infectious diseases

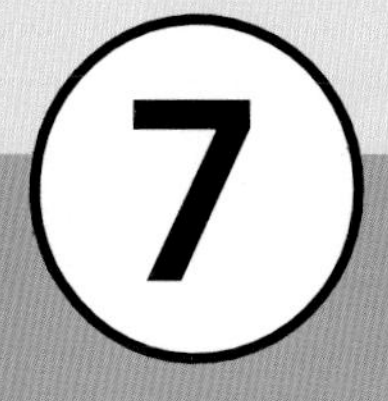

# Respiratory infections

## 7.1 UPPER RESPIRATORY TRACT INFECTIONS

### ACUTE OTITIS MEDIA

- **Key features**: infants are particularly prone owing to their short, horizontal and poorly functioning Eustachian tubes.
- **Infective agents**:
  - **Viral** (50% cases): commonly respiratory syncytial virus (RSV).
  - **Bacterial**:
    - *Haemophilus influenzae*;
    - *Streptococcus pneumoniae*;
    - *Moraxella catarrhalis*;
    - *Streptococcus pyogenes*;
    - *Staphylococcus aureus.*
- **Clinical features**:
  - pain in the affected ear (often spreading to the jaw);
  - fever;
  - irritability;
  - red and bulging tympanic membrane and rupture with pus discharge.
- **Complications**:
  - **Otitis media with effusion (glue ear)**: can cause a conductive hearing loss that can have an impact on a child's speech and language development.
- **Diagnosis**: clinical or microscopy, culture and sensitivity (MC&S) of specimen.
- **Treatment**:
  - **Pain relief**: ibuprofen or paracetamol-based solutions.
  - **Antibiotics**: amoxicillin or erythromycin (penicillin allergy).
  - **Otitis media with effusion**: grommets.

> **MICRO-facts**
>
> **Pulling at the ears** can be a sign of **otitis media** in infants.

## SINUSITIS

- **Key features**: maxillary sinuses most commonly affected.
- **Infective agents**:
  - **Viral**:
    - rhinovirus;
    - influenza virus;
    - parainfluenza virus.
  - **Bacterial**:
    - *S. pneumoniae*;
    - *S. aureus*;
    - *H. influenzae*;
    - *M. catarrhalis*.
- **Clinical features**:
  - nasal discharge;
  - facial pain (over maxillary and frontal sinuses);
  - headache.
- **Complications**: orbital cellulitis.
- **Diagnosis**: sinus aspiration or swab and MC&S (chronic infections only).
- **Treatment**: decongestant sprays and analgesia.

## ACUTE CORYZA (COMMON COLD)

- **Key features**: very common.
- **Infective agents**:
  - **Viral**:
    - rhinoviruses;
    - coronaviruses;
    - RSV.
- **Diagnosis**: clinical.
- **Treatment**: analgesia.

## PHARYNGITIS AND TONSILLITIS

- **Key features**: 70% caused by viruses.
- **Infective agents**:
  - **Viral**:
    - adenovirus;
    - rhinoviruses;
    - enteroviruses;
    - influenza virus;
    - parainfluenza virus.
  - **Bacterial**:
    - *S. pyogenes*;
    - *S. pneumoniae*;

  - *H. influenzae*;
  - *Mycoplasma pneumoniae*.
- **Clinical features**:
  - **Pharyngitis**:
    - sore throat;
    - myalgia;
    - fever;
    - coryzal symptoms.
  - **Tonsillitis**:
    - sore throat;
    - lymphadenopathy;
    - dysphagia;
    - malaise;
    - exudate on soft palate.
  - **Scarlet fever**: *S. pyogenes* sore throat with an erythematous rash and strawberry red tongue owing to toxin production.
- **Complications**:
  - Peri-tonsillar (quinsy) and retropharyngeal abscesses.
  - **Group A *Streptococcus***: post-infective rheumatic fever and glomerulonephritis.
- **Diagnosis**: clinical.
- **Treatment**:
  - **Severe cases**: phenoxymethylpenicillin (penicillin V) or erythromycin (penicillin allergy).
  - **Analgesia**: aspirin gargle or paracetamol.

## INFECTIOUS MONONUCLEOSIS (GLANDULAR FEVER)

- **Key features**: the symptoms of glandular fever are caused by the immune response to the Epstein–Barr virus as opposed to a direct pathogenic effect of the virus.
- **Infective agents**:
  - **Viral**: Epstein–Barr virus.
- **Clinical features**:
  - sore throat;
  - fever;
  - petechiae on soft palate;
  - lymphadenopathy (cervical);
  - hepatosplenomegaly;
  - coryzal symptoms.
- **Complications**:
  - airway obstruction owing to enlarged tonsils;
  - post-infective chronic fatigue or depression.

- **Diagnosis**:
  - Immunoglobulin (Ig) M antibody to virus capsid antigen (gold standard).
  - Lymphocytosis.
  - **Blood film**: atypical enlarged lymphocytes.
  - Monospot test.
- **Treatment**: analgesia (e.g. aspirin gargle or paracetamol).

> **MICRO-facts**
>
> The **monospot test** detects **Epstein–Barr virus antibodies** but has **low sensitivity** with **young children**.
>
> **Amoxicillin** may provoke a **maculopapular rash** with **infectious mononucleosis**.

## ACUTE EPIGLOTTITIS

- **Key features**: occurs mainly in children less than 6 years old.
- **Infective agents**: *H. influenzae* (type b).
- **Clinical features**:
  - rapid onset, patient becomes very unwell;
  - high fever (greater than 38.5°C);
  - painful throat causes the child to drool saliva and be reluctant to talk, eat or drink;
  - soft stridor.
- **Complications**: bacteraemia.
- **Diagnosis**: clinical.
- **Treatment**:
  - Contact a senior anaesthetist, paediatrician and ENT surgeon.
  - Intubation under general anaesthetic or tracheostomy if intubation not possible.
  - **Antibiotics**: cefotaxime or chloramphenicol.
  - **Close contact prophylaxis**: rifampicin for household contacts.
  - **Immunization (UK schedule)**: 2, 3, 4 and 12 months.

> **MICRO-facts**
>
> If epiglottitis is suspected DO NOT:
>
> **examine** the throat with a **spatula**;
>
> **lie** the patient **down**;
>
> cause unnecessary **distress**.
>
> These can all cause the **airway** to **constrict** and obstruct.

### ACUTE LARYNGOTRACHEOBRONCHITIS (CROUP)

- **Key features**: occurs mainly in children aged 6 months to 6 years.
- **Infective agents**:
  - parainfluenza virus;
  - RSV (rarely).
- **Clinical features**:
  - onset over days with coryzal symptoms;
  - barking cough;
  - fever;
  - harsh stridor.
- **Diagnosis**: clinical.
- **Treatment**: inhalation of moist air or dexamethasone (severe disease with airway obstruction).

### BACTERIAL TRACHEITIS (PSEUDOMEMBRANOUS CROUP)

- **Key features**: can follow intubation.
- **Infective agents**:
  - *S. aureus*;
  - *H. influenzae*.
- **Clinical features**: similar to acute epiglottitis.
- **Diagnosis**: clinical.
- **Treatment**: flucloxacillin (for *S. aureus*) or cephalosporin.

## 7.2 PNEUMONIA

### DEFINITION

- An acute infection of the lower respiratory tract.

### CLASSIFICATION AND INFECTIVE AGENTS

- See Table 7.1

### SYMPTOMS

- **Systemic**: fever, myalgia, arthralgia, rigors and headache.
- **Respiratory**:
  - cough;
  - dyspnoea;
  - pleuritic chest pain.

### SIGNS

- **Consolidation**:
  - reduced chest expansion on affected side;

Table 7.1 Classification of pneumonia and infective agents

| | COMMUNITY ACQUIRED | HOSPITAL ACQUIRED (NOSOCOMIAL) | ASPIRATION | IMMUNO-COMPROMISED | ATYPICAL | CHILDHOOD |
|---|---|---|---|---|---|---|
| Definition | Develop as outpatient or within 48 hours of hospital admission | Develops atleast 48 hours after hospital admission | Inhalation of gastric contents resulting in infection | Increased risk of pneumonia due to underlying disease, e.g. HIV/AIDS, leukaemia | Pneumonia associated with specific organisms | Pneumonia during childhood |
| Organisms | *Streptococcus pneumoniae* (most common) | Gram-negative bacilli, e.g. *Escherichia coli* and *Klesbsiella pneumoniae* | *Streptococcus pneumoniae* | *Streptococcus pneumoniae* (post-splenectomy) | *Mycoplasma pneumoniae* | **Neonates**: *Streptococcus agalactiae* *Escherichia coli* *Chlamydia trachomatis* |
| | *Haemophilus influenzae* | *Pseudomonas aeruginosa* | Anaerobes | *Haemophilus influenzae* | *Legionella pneumophila* | |
| | *Mycoplasma pneumoniae* | *Staphylococcus aureus* | Gram-negative bacilli, e.g. *Escherichia coli* and *Klesbsiella pneumoniae* | *Staphylococcus aureus* | *Chlamydophila pneumoniae* | **Infants**: *Streptococcus pneumoniae* *Staphylococcus aureus* *Haemophilus influenzae* RSV Adenoviruses |
| | *Staphylococcus aureus* | | | Gram-negative bacilli | *Chlamydophila psittaci* | |

Table 7.1 (*continued*)

| | COMMUNITY ACQUIRED | HOSPITAL ACQUIRED (NOSOCOMIAL) | ASPIRATION | IMMUNO-COMPROMISED | ATYPICAL | CHILDHOOD |
|---|---|---|---|---|---|---|
| | *Chlamydophila pneumoniae* | | | **Viruses**: CMV and HSV | *Coxiella burnetii* (Q-fever) | **Children**: *Streptococcus pneumoniae* *Haemophilus influenzae* *Streptococcus pyogenes* |
| | Influenza A (usually with bacterial infection) | | | **Fungi**: *Pneumocystis jiroveci*, *Cryptococcus* spp. and *Histoplasma* spp. | | |

AIDS, acquired immune deficiency syndrome; CMV, cytomegalovirus; HIV, human immunodeficiency virus; HSV, herpes simplex virus; RSV, respiratory syncytial virus.

  - dull percussion note over infected area;
  - bronchial breathing;
  - crackles;
  - increased tactile vocal fremitus and vocal resonance.
- **Respiratory**:
  - tachypnoea;
  - tachycardia;
  - cyanosis.

## SPECIFIC PNEUMONIAS

- ***Mycoplasma pneumoniae***:
  - More common in younger patients (second and third decade).
  - Outbreaks occur every 3–4 years.
  - **Clinical features**: flu-like illness for 1–5 days followed by dry cough.
  - **Extrapulmonary complications**:
    - **Skin**: erythema multiforme and Stevens–Johnson syndrome.
    - **Haematological**: autoimmune haemolytic anaemia (cold type).
    - **Cardiac**: pericarditis and myocarditis.
    - **Neurological**: meningoencephalitis.
  - **Investigations**: uni/bilateral consolidation on chest radiograph and antibody serology.
- ***Legionella pneumophila***:
  - Outbreaks commonly among fit patients staying at hotels or institutions with contaminated water tanks (less than 60°C).
  - **Clinical features**: flu-like illness before developing a dry cough and shortness of breath.
  - **Extrapulmonary complications**:
    - **Renal**: renal failure.
    - **Gastrointestinal**: diarrhoea, vomiting and hepatitis.
    - **Neurological**: confusion and coma.
  - **Investigations**: lobar or multilobar shadowing on chest radiograph, hyponatraemia and lymphocytopenia and antigen testing (serum and urinary).
- ***Coxiella burnetii* (Q-fever)**:
  - Typically affects livestock (sheep, cattle and goats) and is transferred via urine, faeces, milk and within the placenta.
  - **Clinical features**: flu-like illness with high temperature and dry cough. Endocarditis and hepatitis can develop.
  - **Chronic infection**: associated with endocarditis, uveitis and osteomyelitis.
  - **Investigations**: serological antibody testing.
- ***Chlamydia psittaci* (psittacosis)**:
  - Linked with exposure to infected birds (such as parrots), although this is not always true.

- **Clinical features**: flu-like illness and dry cough or high temperature, photophobia and neck stiffness (appears similar to meningitis).
- **Investigations**: rising antibody titre.

- ***Klebsiella pneumoniae***:
  - Associated with older patients, diabetes mellitus and alcoholism.
  - **Clinical features**: sudden onset, flu-like illness, high fever and productive cough with blood-tinged sputum (red currant jelly sputum).
- ***Pneumocystis jiroveci* (*carinii*; formerly known as *Pneumocystis carinii* pneumonia (PCP))**:
  - Associated with immunosuppression, typically human immunodeficiency virus (HIV)/acquired immune deficiency syndrome (AIDS) infection.
  - **Clinical features**: dry cough, dyspnoea and high fever.
  - **Investigations**: diffuse bilateral interstitial perihilar shadowing on chest radiograph and sputum staining from bronchoalveolar lavage or induced sputum techniques (e.g. nebulized hypertonic saline).
  - Patients with HIV/AIDS should receive co-trimoxazole prophylaxis when their $CD4^+$ count is less than 200 cells/$mm^3$.
  - All patients diagnosed with PCP should be counselled for HIV testing.

## INVESTIGATIONS

- **Sputum**: for MC&S.
- **Urinary antigens**: *L. pneumophila* and *M. pneumoniae.*
- **Bloods**:
  - **Full blood count**: raised white cell count and neutrophilia.
  - **Urea and electrolytes**: urea levels are a useful prognostic factor (see below).
  - Liver function tests.
  - C-reactive protein/erythrocyte sedimentation rate (ESR).
  - Blood cultures.
- **Serology**: atypical organisms (see above).
- **Chest radiograph**:
  - consolidation (lags behind presenting features by up to 2 days);
  - pleural effusion.

## MANAGEMENT

- **Severity**: assess using CURB-65 score:
  - **C** = confusion ($<8$ on the abbreviated mental test);
  - **U** = urea $>7$ mmol/L;
  - **R** = respiratory rate $>30$/min;
  - **B** = blood pressure $<90$ systolic or diastolic $\leq 60$;
  - **65** = age $\geq$ 65 years old.

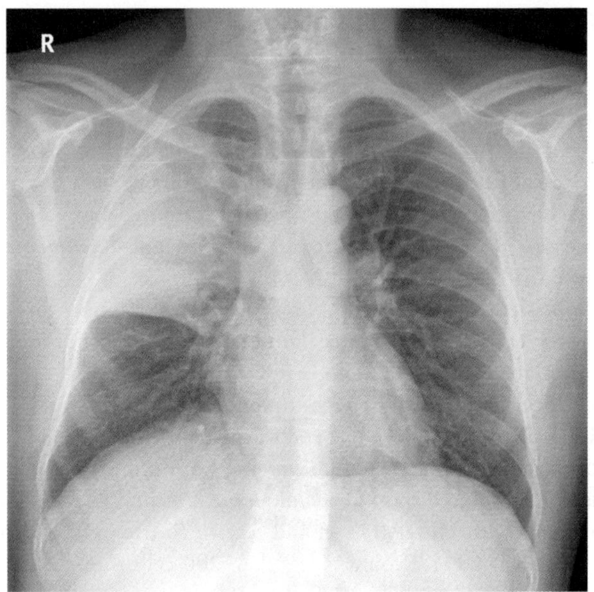


Fig. 7.1 Chest radiograph showing right upper lobe pneumonia. Courtesy of Dr I. Bickle, Northern General Hospital, Sheffield, UK.

- **Score**:
  - **0–1**: home treatment;
  - **2**: hospital therapy;
  - **3 +** : severe pneumonia.
- **Medication**:
  - **Mild uncomplicated community acquired**: amoxicillin or erythromycin (penicillin allergy).
  - **Severe community acquired**: co-amoxiclav or cefuroxime and erythromycin.
  - **Hospital acquired**:
    - **Gram-negative bacilli**: gentamicin and third-generation cephalosporin.
    - ***Pseudomonas* spp.**: ciprofloxacin or piperacillin and tazobactam or ceftazidime.
  - **Aspiration**: metronidazole and cefuroxime.
  - **Atypical**:
    - ***Legionella* spp**.: clarithromycin or ciprofloxacin or rifampicin (severe cases).
    - ***Chlamydia* spp**.: doxycycline.
    - ***P. jiroveci* (formerly*P. carinii*)**: co-trimoxazole.

### COMPLICATIONS

- **Respiratory**:
  - **Pleural effusion**: exudative effusion which may worsen breathing symptoms and cause chest pain.
  - **Empyema**: pus in the pleural space, appears similar to pleural effusion on radiograph. Treat with a chest drain or decortication.
  - **Lung abscess**:
    - Pus-filled cavity within the lung.
    - Typically with aspiration pneumonia or poorly treated cases.
    - **Clinical features**: persisting pneumonia, copious foul-smelling sputum, swinging fevers, weight loss and clubbing.
    - **Investigations**: anaemia, raised ESR and cavity on chest radiograph.
- **Cardiovascular**:
  - **Septicaemia**: can cause sudden deterioration and haematogenous spread (e.g. meningitis, endocarditis or pericarditis).
  - **Hypotension**: associated with septic vasodilatation.
  - Atrial fibrillation.

**MICRO-reference**

British Thoracic Society. *Guidelines for the management of community acquired pneumonia in adults.* Update 2009. A Quick Reference Guide. London, UK: BTS, 2009. Available from: http://www.brit-thoracic.org.uk/Portals/0/Clinical%20Information/Pneumonia/Guidelines/CAPGuideline-full.pdf

## 7.3 OTHER LOWER RESPIRATORY TRACT INFECTIONS

### BRONCHIOLITIS

- **Key features**:
  - most common in infants less than 1 year old;
  - infants with bronchopulmonary dysplasia or congenital heart disease are at high risk.
- **Infective agents**:
  - **Viral**:
    - RSV (most commonly);
    - parainfluenza virus;
    - human metapneumovirus;
    - adenovirus.

- **Clinical features**:
  - **Initially**: coryzal symptoms.
  - **Later**: wheeze and shortness of breath (causes feeding difficulties).
  - Dry cough.
  - Subcostal and intercostal recessions.
  - Fine end-inspiratory crackles.
- **Complications**:
  - **Non-atopic wheezing**: episodes of wheezing during childhood in the absence of atopy.
  - **Bronchiolitis obliterans**: granulation tissue is deposited in the bronchioles causing chronic respiratory damage.
- **Diagnosis**:
  - **Nasopharyngeal aspirate**: viral culture or immunofluorescence for RSV.
  - **Chest radiograph**: rarely used in suspected bronchiolitis but may show hyperinflation and exclude differential diagnoses.
- **Treatment**:
  - **Supportive**: humidified oxygen, nutrition and fluid support.
  - **Palivizumab**: monoclonal antibody, reduces severity of RSV illness but reserved for children with congenital immunodeficiency or chronic lung disease.

## WHOOPING COUGH

- **Key features**:
  - uncommon in the UK since vaccination scheme started in the 1950s;
  - significant cause of infant mortality globally.
- **Infective agents**: *Bordetella pertussis.*
- **Clinical features**:
  - **Catarrhal stage**: sneezing, cough and conjunctivitis.
  - **Paroxysmal stage**: severe cough with inspiratory 'whoop' sound and subsequent subconjunctival haemorrhages.
  - **Convalescent stage**: coughing becomes less severe over several months.
- **Diagnosis**: nasal swab for culture.
- **Treatment**: erythromycin or clarithromycin.

**MICRO-case**

Mr B is a 62-year-old painter and decorator on holiday with his partner in Corfu. He visits the local hospital after a week away from home, as he has had a worsening dry cough with sporadic high temperatures over the past week. He explains to the doctor that he decided to visit hospital today as the cough has become productive and he developed diarrhoea last night. He feels tired and achy.

*continued...*

*continued...*

The doctor sends off blood samples to test his electrolytes and full blood count and sends a sputum sample for microscopy. She also orders a chest radiograph.

The microscopy results for the sputum are negative. The chest radiograph shows lobar shadowing and a small right-sided pleural effusion. The blood samples reveal lymphopenia and hyponatraemia.

Not happy with the sputum results, the doctor rings the laboratory, giving clinical details, and is told to send another sample that they will stain with an immunofluorescent stain. She also obtains a urine sample, which is tested for *Legionella* antigen.

The sputum sample reveals a Gram-negative organism – *Legionella pneumophila* – and the urine test is positive. During Mr B's admission, others from the hotel he has been staying in are admitted with similar symptoms. The hotel is found to have *L. pneumophila* contaminating the shower heads and is temporarily closed while the water system is decontaminated.

Mr B is given clarithromycin and recovers completely, returning home a week later.

**Points to consider**:

- *L. pneumophila* is a common cause of sporadic outbreaks of pneumonia in institutions such as hotels, as it can contaminate shower systems.
- *L. pneumophila* often affects previously healthy people, but when the elderly are affected it can be fatal.
- When sending specimens to the laboratory, make sure clinical details are sent with the specimen to ensure that the microbiologists can undertake appropriate tests. If you are unsure which tests to order, ask someone!

## 7.4 TUBERCULOSIS

### EPIDEMIOLOGY

- It is estimated that one-third of the world's population is infected with tuberculosis (TB).
- Globally, TB is the second most fatal infectious disease, behind HIV/AIDS.
- India, China, Indonesia, Bangladesh and Pakistan share more than half of the global burden of TB.
- TB is characterized as a disease of the poor, favouring overcrowded and impoverished environments.

### INFECTIVE AGENTS

- **TB complex**:
  - ***Mycobacterium tuberculosis***: most common cause in humans.
  - ***Mycobacterium bovis***: common among cattle; infection can spread through unpasteurized milk.
  - ***Mycobacterium africanum***: prevalent in equatorial Africa.

## PATHOPHYSIOLOGY

- **Transmission**:
  - airborne droplet nuclei containing *M. tuberculosis* produced by coughing, sneezing and talking during active pulmonary TB infection;
  - small droplet size means that *M. tuberculosis* can be airborne for minutes to hours;
  - infective droplet inhaled into alveoli.
- **Primary infection**:
  - *M. tuberculosis* is taken up by alveolar macrophages. Subsequently, two processes can occur: disease containment (latent TB infection) or active disease (10%) (progressive primary TB or post-primary TB).
    - **Disease containment (latent TB infection)**:
      - *M. tuberculosis* replicates within macrophage;
      - spreads via the lymphatic system to hilar lymph nodes;
      - cell-mediated immunity (2–8/52 post-infection) causes activation of T lymphocytes (mainly $CD4^+$ cells) and macrophages;
      - T lymphocytes and macrophages contain *M. tuberculosis* within a central granuloma (Ghon complex) that is necrotic, caseating and enclosed by epithelioid histiocytes, Langhans' giant cells and lymphocytes;
      - granulomas usually heal in the immunocompetent;
      - dormant *M. tuberculosis* within the granuloma can remain viable and reactivate at a later date (post-primary TB).
    - **Active disease (progressive primary or post-primary TB)**:
      - Active TB disease may occur with the initial infection (progressive primary TB) or as a result of a reactivation of *Mycobacteria* in the Ghon complex (post-primary TB).
      - **Risk factors**: children less than 5 years old or advanced immunosuppression.

## SYMPTOMS (PRIMARY INFECTION AND PULMONARY TUBERCULOSIS)

- TB can affect any organ (spread via lymphatics or bloodstream), but the lung parenchyma is the most commonly affected site in adults as this is the initial site of infection.
- **Primary infection**:
  - **Immunocompetent**: usually asymptomatic; 10% with symptoms develop progressive primary TB.
  - **Immunocompromised/children**: fever, cough and dyspnoea.
- **Progressive primary TB/post-primary TB**:
  - **Systemic**:
    - fever;
    - weight loss;

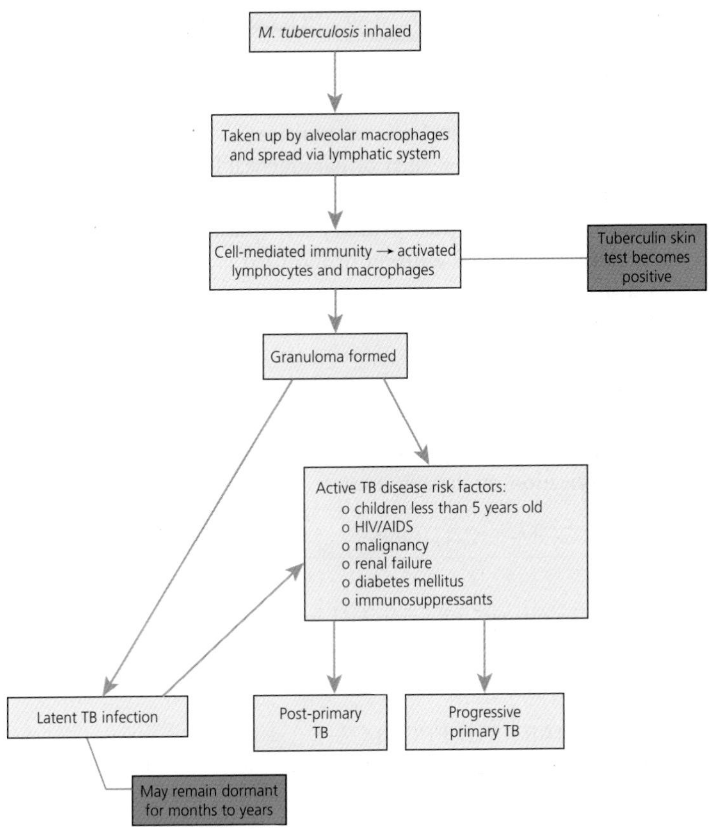


Fig. 7.2 Flowchart showing the pathophysiology of *Mycobacterium tuberculosis*. AIDS, acquired immune deficiency syndrome; HIV, human immunodeficiency virus; TB, tuberculosis.

  - night sweats;
  - malaise.
- **Respiratory**:
  - cough (more than 2–3 weeks, often unproductive);
  - haemoptysis;
  - chest pain (usually pleuritic);
  - dyspnoea.

## MICRO-facts

Pulmonary tuberculosis can appear similar to sarcoidosis with dyspnoea, erythema nodosum, granuloma and bilateral hilar lymphadenopathy.

## SIGNS (PRIMARY INFECTION AND PULMONARY TUBERCULOSIS)

- **Primary infection**:
  - **Erythema nodosum**: painful red/purple nodules on shins.
  - **Tuberculin skin test**: becomes positive.
  - **Chest radiograph**: ± hilar or paratracheal lymphadenopathy ± lung consolidation.
- **Progressive primary TB/post-primary TB (pulmonary)**:
  - **Respiratory**: pleural effusion or localized crackles.
  - **Cardiac**: tachycardia.
  - **Hands**: clubbing (prolonged pulmonary TB can cause bronchiectasis).
  - **Chest radiograph**:
    - consolidation;
    - cavitation;
    - fibrosis (usually upper lobes);
    - calcification in chronic disease.

## PULMONARY COMPLICATIONS

- **TB pleurisy**:
  - Occurs in primary infection and post-primary TB.
  - **Symptoms**: pleuritic chest pain, fever and dry cough.
- **Empyema**: following rupture of TB cavity.

## EXTRAPULMONARY TUBERCULOSIS

- **TB lymphadenitis**:
  - unilateral;
  - chronic (weeks to months);
  - enlarge/discharge during TB treatment (compared with HIV lymphadenopathy, which is persistent and generalized).
- **Central nervous system TB**:
  - **Meningitis**:
    - **Symptoms**: headache, fever, cranial nerve palsies, altered consciousness, fits and coma.
    - Slow onset.
    - Generally fatal without medication (anti-TB medication and corticosteroids).
    - More common in children and immunosuppressed.
  - **Tuberculomas**: space-occupying lesion.
- **Genitourinary TB**:
  - Renal parenchymal destruction causes urethral strictures and bladder shrinkage.
  - **Symptoms**: dysuria, frequency, haematuria and flank pain.

   - **Investigations**: MC&S of three early morning urine samples will show sterile pyuria. *M. tuberculosis* can be cultured from these samples but pick-up rates are low.
   - **Male manifestations**:
     - prostatitis;
     - epididymo-orchitis;
     - painless scrotal mass.
   - **Female manifestations**
     - endometritis and salpingitis (may cause infertility).
- **Gastrointestinal TB**:
   - **Ileitis**:
     - May accompany pulmonary TB.
     - Terminal ileum most common site.
     - **Symptoms**: weight loss, anorexia, abdominal pain and altered bowel habit.
     - **Complications**: fistula, bowel perforation and obstruction.
   - **Peritoneal TB**:
     - **Symptoms**: fever, weight loss, abdominal swelling and irregular bowel habit.
- **Bone TB**:
   - **Pott's disease**: vertebral column TB (most commonly affected bony structure; also large joints, including hip, knee and shoulder).
     - **Symptoms**: back pain, fever and weight loss.
     - **Complications**: paravertebral/psoas abscesses, kyphosis and paraplegia.
- **Cardiovascular TB**:
   - **Pericarditis**:
     - May accompany pulmonary TB.
     - **Symptoms**: pericardial pain.
     - **Signs**: pericardial rub.
     - **Complications**: pericardial effusion and tamponade.
- **Disseminated TB**:
   - TB infection of many organs simultaneously.
   - Most common in children with progressive primary TB and patients with post-primary TB.
   - **Miliary TB**: millet seed-sized lesions (2–4 mm on radiograph) seen in organs with high blood flow (e.g. lungs and bone marrow).

## INVESTIGATIONS

- **Sputum sample**:
   - if cough has lasted longer than 2–3 weeks;
   - three samples for microscopy for acid-fast bacilli and *M. tuberculosis* culture and sensitivities;

    - if no spontaneous samples, sputum may be induced with saline and salbutamol nebulizers;
    - bronchoalveolar lavage is an option if induced sputum is negative for acid-fast bacilli on microscopy.
- **Fluid sample**:
    - **Examples**:
        - early morning urine sample;
        - pleural fluid from a pleural effusion;
        - ascitic fluid;
        - tuberculosis blood cultures (special culture medium required).
    - Low culture yield compared with tissue or sputum samples.

> **MICRO-facts**
>
> Any sample for **suspected tuberculosis** will be immediately examined for **acid-fast bacilli** and then **cultured** to **identify** the **type**.

- **Histology**:
    - Extrapulmonary tissue samples (e.g. pleural or lymph node biopsy).
    - **Characteristic features**: acid-fast bacilli, caseating granulomata with cells derived from macrophages, including epithelioid and multinucleate (Langhans) giant cells.
    - Tissue samples can be cultured for *M. tuberculosis* (higher yield than fluid samples).
- **Chest radiograph**:
    - Characteristic features: consolidation, cavitation and calcification.
    - Not commonly used as non-specific.
    - May exclude pulmonary TB if normal.
- **Interferon-γ release assays (IGRAs)**:
    - T cells sensitized to *M. tuberculosis* will secrete interferon γ (IFN-γ) when re-exposed to *M. tuberculosis* antigens.
    - A variety of test kits (including Quantiferon and T-Spot) can rapidly detect the rise in IFN-γ using a peripheral blood sample.
    - Cannot differentiate between latent and active infection.
- **Tuberculin skin test** (also known as the Mantoux test):
    - Intradermal injection of a TB antigen with review of site at 48–72 hours for reaction between antigen and host TB antibodies.
    - **Positive result (red skin reaction)**: active infection (strong reaction) or immunity (through bacille Calmette–Guérin (BCG) immunization or previous infection).

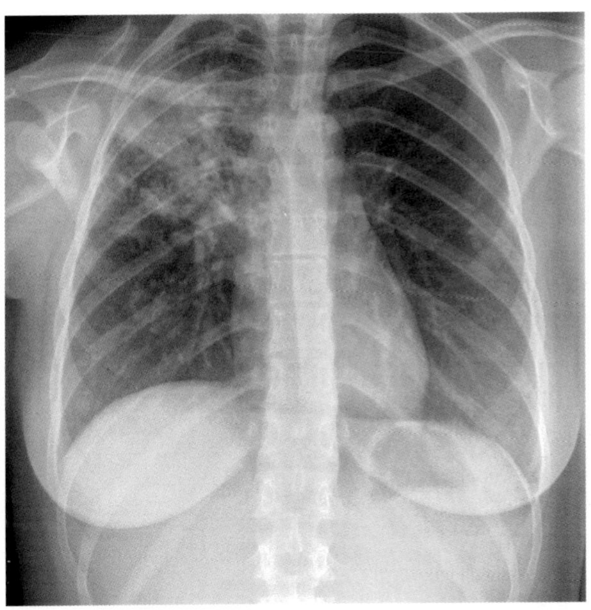

Fig. 7.3 Chest radiograph showing pulmonary tuberculosis infection. Courtesy of Dr I. Bickle, Northern General Hospital, Sheffield, UK.

- **False negatives**: immunosuppression, severe TB (e.g. miliary TB) or incorrect technique.

> **MICRO-facts**
>
> Following cell-mediated activation, the tuberculin skin test and **interferon-$\gamma$ release assays** become positive.

## MANAGEMENT

- Rapid liquid culture can confirm diagnosis in 7–10 days whereas acid-fast bacilli cultures can take up to 12 weeks.
- Anti-tuberculosis therapy should be started immediately if the diagnosis is suspected.
- Most treatment regimens have two phases:
  - **Initial intensive phase**:
    - **Aim**: kill active *Mycobacteria* spp. and reduce chance of resistance.
    - Rifampicin, isoniazid, ethambutol and pyrazinamide for 8 weeks.

- **Continuation phase**:
  - **Aim**: eliminate residual *Mycobacteria* spp.
  - Rifampicin and isoniazid for a further 16 weeks.
- **Infection control**:
  - Patients suspected of active pulmonary TB with a cough should wear a facemask in public areas.
  - Patients should be nursed in a side room, ideally with negative pressure to prevent transmission.
  - All staff and visitors should wear a facemask when in contact with the patient.

> **MICRO-facts**
>
> Major side-effects of tuberculosis **treatment**:
>
> **Rifampicin**: hepatotoxicity.
>
> **Isoniazid**: peripheral neuropathy (start pyridoxine (vitamin B6) at same time to prevent).
>
> **Ethambutol**: ocular toxicity.
>
> **Pyrazinamide**: hepatotoxicity.

## DRUG-RESISTANT TUBERCULOSIS

- *M. tuberculosis* has become increasingly resistant to anti-TB medications:
  - **Multiple drug-resistant TB (MDR-TB)**: resistant to isoniazid and rifampicin (± other drugs).
  - **Extremely drug-resistant TB (XDR-TB)**: MDR-TB and resistance to ciprofloxacin and at least one injectable antibiotic.
- These trends, in combination with little pharmaceutical investment in anti-TB medications, represent a significant threat to global TB control.

> **MICRO-facts**
>
> **Tuberculosis** is a **notifiable disease** in the **UK**.

## PREVENTION

- **BCG immunization**:
  - Live attenuated strain of *M. bovis*.
  - No longer part of UK immunization schedule; reserved only for high-risk groups such as those with close family members from high-risk areas.
  - Can be given at any age.
  - **Contraindications**: HIV/AIDS and malignancy.

**MICRO-reference**

National Institute for Health and Clinical Excellence. *Clinical diagnosis and management of tuberculosis, and measures for its prevention and control.* Clinical Guidance 33. London, UK: NICE, 2006. Available from: http: //guidance.nice.org.uk/CG33

**MICRO-case**

Miss H is a 32 year old who has been on methadone for 3 months after using intravenous drugs for 10 years. She presents to her GP with gradually increasing tiredness and weight loss, which she initially put down to the methadone and coming off drugs, but is now becoming concerned. She also has a productive cough, which is occasionally flecked with blood.

On examination, her chest is clear and all else appears normal. On weighing Miss H, the doctor finds she has lost almost a stone since he saw her last month. The doctor orders a chest radiograph and sends a sputum sample. He also counsels her and advises her to get human immunodeficiency virus (HIV) and hepatitis B and C tests at the genitourinary medicine (GUM) clinic.

The sputum sample comes back confirming *Mycobacteria tuberculosis* infection and the chest radiograph shows patchy shadowing in the upper zones and multiple cavitating lesions. The tests at the GUM clinic all come back negative.

Miss H is started on a 2 month regime of rifampicin, isoniazid, pyrazinamide and ethambutol followed by 4 months of rifampicin and isoniazid. All close contacts are tested with the tuberculin skin test and a radiograph.

Miss H goes back to her GP the next week worried that there is blood in her urine. The doctor tests her urine and reassures her that it is the rifampicin which is dying her urine an orange colour. However, 2 months later she appears to have made very little improvement owing to poor compliance with her drugs. She is entered into the directly observed short course, where she is supervised taking her medication and improves dramatically.

**Points to note**:

- Tuberculosis (TB) is on the increase in developed countries and must be considered even in patients who have had a bacille Calmette–Guérin vaccination.
- TB is very common in HIV-positive patients and HIV should be excluded.
- Patients must be correctly counselled on potential side-effects of the drugs to try and improve compliance.

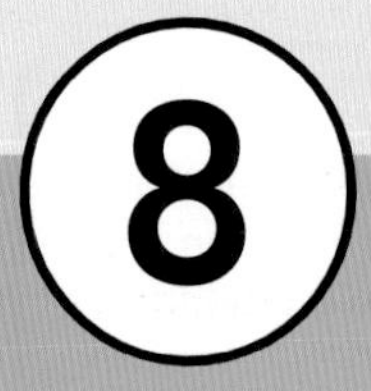


# Gastrointestinal infections

## 8.1 INFECTIVE GASTROENTERITIS

**Table 8.1** shows common causes of gastroenteritis with the incubation period, mechanism, duration, transmission route, clinical features, diagnostic methods and treatment options.

> **MICRO-facts**
>
> Infection with *Escherichia coli* O157:H7 can precipitate haemolytic uremic syndrome: 1) haemolytic anaemia; 2) acute renal failure; 3) thrombocytopenia.
>
> **Norovirus**
>
> Occurs in epidemics, particularly in the winter, often affecting nursing homes and hospitals. It is spread by faecal–oral transmission; therefore, infection control measures are essential. Hand-washing should be rigorous, patients should be nursed in a side room and gloves and apron should be worn.
>
> ***Clostridium difficile (C. diff)***
>
> A major infection control problem in hospitals. Broad-spectrum antibiotic use encourages overgrowth of *C. diff* in the gastrointestinal tract, leading to diarrhoea, or, in severe cases, pseudomembranous colitis. Drugs such as ciprofloxacin and cephalosporins are particularly high risk. Its spores are spread by faecal–oral transmission; therefore, infection control measures are essential. Hand-washing should be rigorous, patients should be nursed in a side room and gloves and apron should be worn. Bedside alcohol gel is less effective than hand-washing for *C. diff* infection. Treatment is with intravenous or oral metronidazole or with oral vancomycin.
>
> **Normal flora**
>
> The human gut is one of the most ecodiverse areas anywhere in the world. Normal gut flora compete with each other and prevent overgrowth of any particular species. These micro-organisms are essential for normal bowel and digestive function. *Clostridium difficile* colitis is an example of the normal gut flora balance being upset.
>
> *continued...*

*continued...*

Gut commensals such as *Escherichia coli* become pathogenic only when in excess or when they spread to normally sterile areas of the body, e.g. the peritoneum or urinary tract.

Do not forget **non-infective causes of diarrhoea** such as **inflammatory bowel disease** and **malignancy**.

**MICRO-case**

Mina is a 4 year old from a remote village in the highlands of Papua New Guinea. A visiting health worker sees her with her mother at the monthly clinic. Her mother reports that Mina has had diarrhoea for the past 3 days. She describes the diarrhoea as very profuse, almost like water, with no blood. Mina does not have any pain with it. Through further questioning, it becomes apparent that several other village members have also been unwell recently with similar symptoms. On examination, Mina is tachycardic, with cold, clammy hands and her eyes appear sunken.

Seeing that Mina is so unwell, the health worker takes Mina straight to the nearest hospital, which is 2 hours away. Mina begins to have convulsions.

On arrival at the hospital a stool sample is taken to the laboratory and Mina is started on intravenous rehydration; 2 hours later Mina goes into respiratory arrest and dies.

The laboratory results show that *Vibrio cholerae* is the causative organism. Several others in the village are taken ill. Tetracycline is given to those in the village with symptoms and all others survive the outbreak.

**Points to note**:

- Although gastroenteritis is a mostly minor condition in developed countries, in developing countries it is a huge cause of mortality.
- Any patient with signs of circulatory collapse must be started on rapid intravenous rehydration.
- Convulsions related to diarrhoea are often caused by electrolyte imbalances, especially low sodium or potassium. Potassium imbalances are particularly important to correct as they can cause fatal arrhythmias. Patients with convulsions must be monitored for aspiration of vomit.

  In outbreaks of cholera, the World Health Organization recommends immunization and/or prophylaxis with tetracycline.
- Education on good hygiene, ensuring clean water supplies and improvement of sanitation are the most effective means of prevention and should be prioritized wherever possible.

Table 8.1 **Gastroenteritis causes, incubation period, duration, transmission, clinical features and treatment**

| PATHOGEN | INCUBATION | MECHANISM | DURATION | TRANSMISSION | SYMPTOMS AND DIAGNOSIS | TREATMENT |
|---|---|---|---|---|---|---|
| **Bacteria** | | | | | | |
| *Staphylococcus aureus* | 2–4 hours (toxin preformed → rapid onset) | Enterotoxin B → intestinal fluid secretion | 24 hours | • Food borne<br>• Poor food hygiene, e.g. food handler with infected hand lesion | • Initially vomiting and abdominal pain; later diarrhoea<br>• Dehydration<br>• **Diagnosis**: culture from vomit or food | • Fluid replacement<br>• Supportive |
| *Shigella* spp. | 1–2 days | Mucosal cell invasion and destruction → diarrhoea with blood and abdominal pain | 5–7 days | • Faecal–oral<br>• Small number of organisms can cause illness | • Dysentery (diarrhoea with blood and mucus)<br>• Fever and abdominal pain<br>• **Complications**: toxic megacolon (rare) and HUS<br>• **Diagnosis**: stool culture | • Fluid replacement<br>• Supportive<br>• Ciprofloxacin or amoxicillin or trimethoprim |
| *Salmonella* spp. | 8–48 hours | Enterotoxin → intestinal fluid secretion | 4–7 days | • Faecal–oral<br>• Commensals of poultry<br>• Contamination of red and white meat, raw eggs and dairy products | • Bloody watery diarrhoea<br>• Nausea and vomiting<br>• Fever<br>• Abdominal pain<br>• Headache<br>• **Diagnosis**: stool or blood culture (rarely used) | • Fluid replacement<br>• Supportive<br>• Ciprofloxacin (decreases severity and duration but rarely used) |

Table 8.1 *(continued)*

| PATHOGEN | INCUBATION | MECHANISM | DURATION | TRANSMISSION | SYMPTOMS AND DIAGNOSIS | TREATMENT |
|---|---|---|---|---|---|---|
| *Campylobacter* spp. | 2–5 days | Mucosal cell invasion and toxin production | 5–7 days | • Faecal–oral<br>• Commensal of livestock<br>• Contamination of undercooked meat (poultry), water and milk | • Diarrhoea (profuse and occasionally bloody)<br>• Nausea and vomiting<br>• Abdominal pain<br>• Fever<br>• **Complications**: Guillain–Barré syndrome<br>• **Diagnosis**: stool culture | • Fluid replacement<br>• Supportive<br>• Erythromycin or azithromycin (severe cases) |
| *Escherichia coli*<br>• Enteroinvasive *E. coli* (EIEC) | • Shigellosis-like disease<br>• **Diagnosis**: stool culture | | | | | |
| • Enterotoxigenic *E. coli* (ETEC) | 1–2 days | Enterotoxin → intestinal fluid secretion | 2–3 days | • Faecal–oral<br>• Contamination of water and food<br>• Common cause of traveller's diarrhoea | • Diarrhoea (watery) | • Fluid replacement<br>• Supportive |
| • Enterohaemorrhagic (EHEC)/verotoxin-producing *E. coli* (VTEC) | 12–48 hours | Serotype O157:H7 secretes Shiga-like toxin 1 → damage of gut and renal endothelial cells | 2–3 days | • Faecal–oral<br>• Contamination of water and food<br>• Commensal of cattle | • Diarrhoea (commonly bloody)<br>• Abdominal pain<br>• Nausea<br>• **Complications**: HUS (7–10 days later)<br>• **Diagnosis**: stool culture | • Fluid replacement<br>• Supportive<br>• HUS: admit to hospital<br>• Avoid antibiotics as may precipitate HUS |

Table 8.1 *(continued)*

| PATHOGEN | INCUBATION | MECHANISM | DURATION | TRANSMISSION | SYMPTOMS AND DIAGNOSIS | TREATMENT |
|---|---|---|---|---|---|---|
| *Vibrio cholerae* | 1–6 days | Enterotoxin → intestinal fluid secretion | $<1$ week | • Faecal–oral<br>• Contamination of water and food<br>• Associated with poor hygiene standards, e.g. refugee camps | • Spectrum of diarrhoeal illness<br>• Mild diarrhoea to profuse watery diarrhoea ($>25$ litres 'rice water' stool per day)<br>• Severe dehydration<br>• **Diagnosis**: clinical, stool culture or microscopy | • Oral/intravenous fluid replacement<br>• Tetracycline reduces time of excretion; therefore, reducing risk of transmission |
| *Clostridium perfringens* | 8–24 hours | Enterotoxin → intestinal fluid secretion | 1 day | • Spores replicate in red/white meat allowed to cool | • Diarrhoea (watery)<br>• Nausea and vomiting<br>• Abdominal pain | • Fluid replacement<br>• Supportive |
| *Clostridium difficile* | Days to months after antibiotics | Enterotoxin (toxin A) → intestinal fluid secretion and cytotoxin (toxin B) → cell damage | Variable | • Normal bowel commensal in 3–5% population<br>• Antibiotics eliminate other bowel flora → *C. difficile* infection<br>• Faecal–oral transmission can occur<br>• Common antibiotics include clindamycin and cephalosporins<br>• Linked to poor hand hygiene in hospitals | • Spectrum of diarrhoeal illness<br>• Mild diarrhoeal illness to pseudomembranous colitis (haemorrhagic colitis, diarrhoea and abdominal pain with colonic pseudomembrane)<br>• Can be fatal in elderly patients<br>• **Diagnosis**: ELISA detection of toxins in stools | • Fluid replacement<br>• Discontinue causative antibiotics<br>• Metronidazole or vancomycin |

Table 8.1 *(continued)*

| PATHOGEN | INCUBATION | MECHANISM | DURATION | TRANSMISSION | SYMPTOMS AND DIAGNOSIS | TREATMENT |
|---|---|---|---|---|---|---|
| *Clostridium botulinum* | 1–2 days | Neurotoxin → paralysis | 2–3 weeks | • Spores contaminate preserved/tinned foods, replicate and produce neurotoxin<br>• Neurotoxin ingested with food | • Diarrhoea<br>• Paralysis<br>• Respiratory muscle paralysis can be fatal<br>• **Diagnosis**: detect toxin in stool sample or food | • Supportive<br>• Antitoxin |
| *Bacillus cereus* | **Vomiting form**: 2–5 hours (toxin preformed)<br>**Diarrhoea form**: 10–12 hours | Produces two toxins → vomiting or diarrhoea | 12–24 hours | • **Vomiting**: spores survive, multiply and produce a toxin in rice left to cool for a long time<br>• **Diarrhoea**: ice cream or meat | • Vomiting<br>• Diarrhoea<br>• Abdominal pain<br>• **Diagnosis**: stool culture | • Fluid replacement<br>• Supportive |
| **Viruses** | | | | | | |
| Rotavirus | 2–3 days | Cell destruction and intestinal fluid secretion | 3–9 days | • Faecal–oral<br>• Environmental contamination<br>• Common in children; adults develop lifelong resistance | • Fever<br>• Vomiting<br>• Diarrhoea<br>• **Diagnosis**: virus isolation in cell culture from stool sample | • Fluid replacement<br>• Supportive |
| Norovirus | 1–2 days | Cell destruction | 1–2 days | • Faecal–oral<br>• Contaminates food, water or environmental surfaces | • Nausea and vomiting<br>• Diarrhoea (watery)<br>• Fever<br>• Headache<br>• Aching limbs | • Fluid replacement<br>• Supportive |

Table 8.1 *(continued)*

| PATHOGEN | INCUBATION | MECHANISM | DURATION | TRANSMISSION | SYMPTOMS AND DIAGNOSIS | TREATMENT |
|---|---|---|---|---|---|---|
| Adenovirus | 3–10 days | Infection of intestinal epithelial cells | 1–2 days | • Faecal–oral | • Diarrhoea<br>• **Diagnosis**: virus isolation in cell culture from stool sample | • Fluid replacement<br>• Supportive |
| **Protozoa** | | | | | | |
| *Giardia lamblia* | 7–21 days | Trophozoites attach to intestinal villi → inflammation | Variable | • Faecal–oral<br>• Cysts contaminate water or food | • Asymptomatic carrier<br>• Diarrhoea (slimy and foul smelling)<br>• Abdominal pain<br>• Nausea and vomiting<br>• Malabsorption<br>• Bloating and excessive flatus<br>• **Diagnosis**: microscopy of stool sample | • Fluid replacement<br>• Supportive<br>• Metronidazole |
| *Cryptosporidium parvum* | 3–6 days | Sporozoites invade intestinal epithelium → inflammation | Several weeks; longer in immunocompromised | • Faecal–oral<br>• Infective cysts contaminate water | • Asymptomatic carrier<br>• Diarrhoea (mild)<br>• More severe disease in immunocompromised patients, typically HIV/AIDS<br>• **Diagnosis**: microscopy of stool sample | • Fluid replacement<br>• Supportive |

Table 8.1 *(continued)*

| PATHOGEN | INCUBATION | MECHANISM | DURATION | TRANSMISSION | SYMPTOMS AND DIAGNOSIS | TREATMENT |
|---|---|---|---|---|---|---|
| *Entamoeba histolytica* | Variable, days to months | Multiplication of trophozoites in the colon can cause inflammation and necrosis | Chronic unless treated | • Faecal–oral.<br>• Infective cysts contaminate water or food | • Chronic mild diarrhoea<br>• Abdominal pain<br>• Later, bloody diarrhoea<br>• Nausea<br>• Headache<br>• **Complications**: toxic megacolon, strictures and liver abscesses<br>• **Diagnosis**: microscopy of stool sample | • Fluid replacement<br>• Supportive<br>• Metronidazole or tinidazole |

AIDS, acquired immune deficiency syndrome; ELISA, enzyme-linked immunosorbent assay; HIV, human immunodeficiency virus; HUS, haemolytic uraemic syndrome.

## 8.2 TYPHOID (ENTERIC FEVER)

### EPIDEMIOLOGY

- More common in developing countries owing to poor sanitation and hygiene.

### INFECTIVE AGENTS

- Typhoid can be caused by two forms of *Salmonella*:
  - *Salmonella typhi*;
  - *Salmonella paratyphi* (types A, B and C).
- Typhoid enteric fever is more severe than paratyphoid enteric fever.

### PATHOPHYSIOLOGY

- **Transmission**:
  - Faecal/urine–oral route (e.g. contaminated food and water).
- **Multiplication and infection**:
  - reduced gastric acid increases susceptibility to *Salmonella* spp.;
  - *Salmonella* spp. penetrate and replicate within epithelial cells and the reticuloendothelial system (macrophages and monocytes);
  - replication can cause a bacteraemia, organ infection and symptoms.
- **Disease progression**:
  - Untreated, 20% die, commonly 2–4 weeks after clinical manifestation.
  - **Causes of death**:
    - encephalopathy;
    - gastrointestinal perforation and haemorrhage (secondary to hypersensitivity reaction in Peyer's patches);
    - peritonitis;
    - toxic myocarditis.

### SYMPTOMS

- **Incubation period**: 10–20 days.
- **Illness duration**: ~4 weeks (untreated cases); symptoms vary with time and tend to improve by week 4.
- **Week 1**:
  - malaise;
  - headache;
  - fever;
  - constipation.
- **Week 2**: high fever.
- **Week 3**:
  - pea soup diarrhoea;
  - coma, delirium and meningism (indicate poor prognosis).

- **Week 4**:
  - Improvement.
  - **Complications**:
    - **Gastrointestinal**: bowel perforation or haemorrhage, hepatitis and chronic cholecystitis (asymptomatic carrier state).
    - **Respiratory**: pneumonia.
    - **Cardiovascular**: pericarditis.
    - **Central nervous system**: meningitis.

## SIGNS

- **Week 2**:
  - bradycardia (relative);
  - hepatosplenomegaly;
  - abdominal distension;
  - rose spots (pink blanching papules found on the trunk).
- **Week 3**: tachypnoea.

## INVESTIGATIONS

- **Cultures**:
  - blood (first 10 days);
  - bone marrow (ideal);
  - urine;
  - stool.
- **Blood tests**:
  - **Liver function tests**: deranged.
  - **Full blood count**: anaemia (due to bleeding).
  - **White cell count**: low.

## MANAGEMENT

- Do not delay treatment as mortality significantly reduced with antibiotics.
- **Antibiotics**: ciprofloxacin (oral or intravenous in severe illness).
- Antibiotic resistance is reported, alternatives include:
  - chloramphenicol (oral);
  - cefotaxime (intravenous);
  - amoxicillin (oral);
  - co-trimoxazole (oral).

## PREVENTION

- Sanitation and hygiene education.
- **Vaccination**:
  - travellers to endemic areas (e.g. South Asia and Africa);
  - laboratory workers at risk of contact with *S. typhi*.

# 8.3 INFECTIVE HEPATITIS

## LIVER INFLAMMATION

- **Non-infective**:
    - drugs;
    - alcohol;
    - autoimmune disease;
    - pregnancy;
    - poisoning.
- **Infective**:
    - Hepatitis A virus.
    - Hepatitis E virus.
    - Hepatitis B virus.
    - Hepatitis D virus.
    - Hepatitis C virus.
    - **Others**: Epstein–Barr virus, cytomegalovirus, yellow fever virus and herpes simplex virus.

## HEPATITIS A VIRUS

- **Key features**:
    - **Viral type**: RNA virus.
    - **Carrier state**: no.
    - **Chronic liver disease**: no.
    - **Hepatocellular cancer**: no.
    - **Mortality**: 0.5%.
    - Most common cause of infective hepatitis.
    - Infection occurs worldwide but is more common in developing countries.
    - Rarely progresses to fulminant hepatitis (liver failure) or cholestatic hepatitis (hepatitis with prolonged jaundice and pruritus).
    - Complete immunity is attained after infection.
- **Transmission**: faecal–oral (e.g. contaminated shellfish, food or water).
- **Incubation period**: 2–6 weeks.
- **Clinical features**:
    - self-limiting;
    - headache;
    - lethargy;
    - nausea;
    - vomiting;
    - jaundice;
    - right upper quadrant pain;
    - anorexia;
    - fever.

- **Diagnosis**:
  - **Liver function tests**: serum transaminases (alanine transaminase (ALT) and aspartate transaminase (AST)) raised and $\gamma$-glutamyl transferase (GGT) normal or raised.
  - **Antibodies**:
    - **Anti-hepatitis A virus (HAV) immunoglobulin (Ig) M**: acute infection.
    - **Anti-HAV IgG**: previous exposure.
- **Treatment**: supportive as self-limiting.
- **Prevention**:
  - **Vaccine**:
    - Inactivated HAV with booster every 10 years.
    - **Suitable groups**:
      - travellers;
      - lifestyle risk;
      - other liver disease.
  - Sanitation and hygiene education.

## HEPATITIS E VIRUS

- **Key features**:
  - **Viral type**: RNA virus.
  - **Carrier state**: no.
  - **Chronic liver disease**: no.
  - **Hepatocellular cancer**: no.
  - **Mortality**: 1–2% (10–20% in pregnancy).
  - Structurally and clinically similar to hepatitis A infection.
  - Often arises in epidemics in developing countries.
- **Transmission**: faecal–oral and transplacentally.
- **Incubation period**: 2–8 weeks.
- **Clinical features**: similar to HAV but generally more severe and higher incidence of progression to liver failure, especially in pregnant women.
- **Diagnosis**:
  - **Liver function tests**: serum transaminases (ALT and AST) raised and GGT normal or raised.
  - **Antibodies**: anti-hepatitis E virus (HEV) IgM.
- **Treatment**: supportive.
- **Prevention**:
  - **Vaccine**: none.
  - Sanitation and hygiene education.

## HEPATITIS B VIRUS

- **Key features**:
  - **Viral type**: deoxyribonucleic acid (DNA) virus.
  - **Carrier state**: yes (potentially asymptomatic).

    - **Chronic liver disease**: yes.
    - **Hepatocellular cancer**: yes.
    - **Mortality**: 1%.
- **Transmission**:
    - blood (needle-stick injuries, sharing needles, blood transfusion with contaminated blood);
    - vertical (most common in the UK);
    - saliva;
    - sexual.
- **Incubation period**: 2–6 months.
- **Clinical features**:
    - similar to HAV (urticaria and arthralgia more common);
    - can be acute and cleared by the immune system (90% adults);
    - may also become chronic (5–10%) or cause hepatocellular carcinoma;
    - often asymptomatic in infants.
- **Serology**:
    - **Antigens**:
        - **Hepatitis B surface antigen (HBsAg)**:
            - acute infection (present in blood 6 weeks to 3 months after acute infection);
            - presence for greater than 6 months signifies chronic hepatitis B infection.
        - **Hepatitis B envelope antigen (HBeAg)**:
            - high level of viral replication and high infectivity.
    - **Antibodies**:
        - **Anti-hepatitis B core antibody (anti-HBc)**:
            - **IgM**: acute viral replication and diagnostic.
            - **IgG + negative HBsAg**: previous exposure.
        - **Anti-hepatitis B surface antibody (anti-HBs)**:
            - hepatitis B immunity (e.g. vaccination).
        - **Anti-hepatitis B envelope antibody (anti-HBe)**:
            - decreased infectivity (absence = high infectivity).

### MICRO-facts

Hepatitis B (HB) serology can be confusing; here is a clinical perspective:

**Acute HB**: hepatitis B surface antigen (HBsAg) and hepatitis B envelope antigen (HBeAg) and anti-hepatitis B core antibody (anti-HBc) immunoglobulin (Ig) M.

**Chronic HB (low infectivity)**: HBsAg (>6/12), anti-hepatitis B envelope antibody (anti-HBe) and anti-HBc IgG.

*continued...*

*continued...*

**Chronic HB (high infectivity)**: HBsAg (>6/12), HBeAg and anti-HBc IgG.

**Cleared infection**: anti-hepatitis B surface antibody (anti-HBs), anti-HBe and anti-HBc IgG.

**Vaccinated**: anti-HBs.

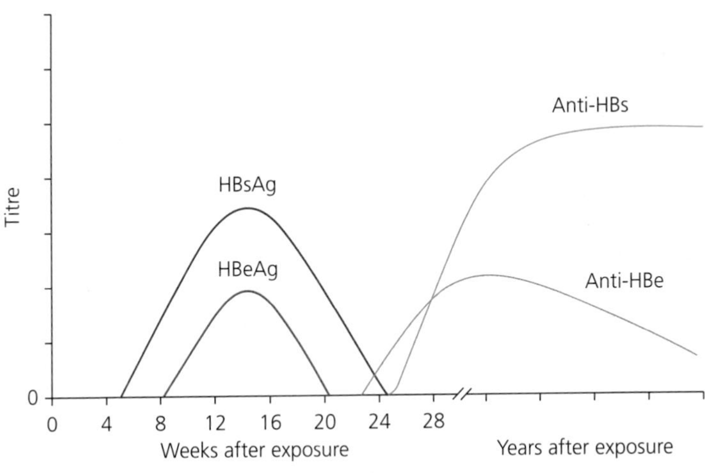


Fig. 8.1 Hepatitis B serology.

- **Diagnosis**:
  - **Liver function tests**: serum transaminases (ALT and AST) raised and GGT normal or raised.
  - See Serology above.
- **Treatment**:
  - Supportive for acute infection.
  - **Chronic infection**:
    - peginterferon alfa-2a;
    - interferon α;
    - adefovir dipivoxil;
    - lamivudine.
  - Monitor treatment response by measuring viral genomic load.
- **Prevention**:
  - **Vaccine**:
    - Inactivated HBsAg.
    - **Suitable groups**:
      - ○ health workers;
      - ○ intravenous drug users and close contacts;

    - babies born to HBV-infected mothers;
    - individuals with chronic liver or renal disease or those receiving regular blood transfusions.

## HEPATITIS D VIRUS

- **Key features**:
    - **Viral type**: RNA virus.
    - **Carrier state**: yes.
    - **Chronic liver disease**: yes.
    - **Hepatocellular cancer**: rare.
    - Only able to infect in the presence of HBV infection (5% co-infected).
- **Transmission**: same as HBV.
- **Incubation period**: 4–12 weeks.
- **Clinical features**:
    - same as HBV;
    - chronic infection with HBV followed by subsequent hepatitis D virus (HDV) infection can lead to accelerated liver failure and cirrhosis.
- **Diagnosis**:
    - **Liver function tests**: serum transaminases (ALT and AST) raised and GGT normal or raised.
    - **Antibodies**: IgM anti-delta antibodies and anti-HBc IgM.
- **Treatment**: as for HBV.
- **Prevention**: as for HBV.

## HEPATITIS C VIRUS

- **Key features**:
    - **Viral type**: RNA virus.
    - **Carrier state**: yes.
    - **Chronic liver disease**: yes.
    - **Hepatocellular cancer**: yes.
    - **Mortality**: 1%.
- **Transmission**:
    - blood (needle-stick injuries, sharing needles, blood transfusion with contaminated blood);
    - vertical;
    - sexual (rarely).
- **Incubation**: 2–26 weeks.
- **Clinical features**:
    - Can be acute and cleared by the immune system (20% adults).
    - May also become chronic (80%) or cause hepatocellular carcinoma.
    - Acute infection often asymptomatic.

- <25% adults become jaundiced.
- **Chronic hepatitis C virus (HCV) infection**:
  - cirrhosis (50%);
  - lymphoma;
  - glomerulonephritis;
  - autoimmune thyroid disease;
  - Raynaud's disease.
- **Diagnosis**:
  - **Liver function tests**: serum transaminases (ALT and AST) raised and GGT normal or raised.
  - **Antibodies**: anti-HCV IgG.
- **Treatment**:
  - pegylated interferon;
  - ribavirin.
- **Prevention**:
  - **Vaccine**: none.
  - Blood products are screened for HCV.
  - Needle exchange programmes and education.

## MICRO-facts

| Virus | Viral type | Carrier state | Chronic liver disease | Hepatocellular carcinoma |
|---|---|---|---|---|
| HAV | RNA | No | No | No |
| HBV | DNA | Yes | Yes | Yes |
| HCV | RNA | Yes | Yes | Yes |
| HDV | RNA | Yes | Yes | Yes, rare |
| HEV | RNA | No | No | No |

HAV, hepatitis A virus; HBV, hepatitis B virus; HCV, hepatitis C virus; HDV, hepatitis D virus; HEV, hepatitis E virus; RNA, ribonucleic acid; DNA, deoxyribonucleic acid.

# 9 Cardiovascular infections

## 9.1 INFECTIVE ENDOCARDITIS

### DEFINITION

- An infection of the endocardial surface of the heart.

### EPIDEMIOLOGY

- More common in men than women.
- Up to half of all cases occur in elderly patients, especially those with co-morbidities such as diabetes.

### INFECTIVE AGENTS

- **Bacteria**:
  - *Staphylococcus aureus* (intravenous drug use (IVDU), indwelling vascular catheters and prosthetic or native valves).
  - Coagulase-negative *Staphylococcus* spp. (neonates and prosthetic heart valves).
  - *Viridans* streptococci (dental conditions or procedures).
  - *Streptococcus agalactiae.*
  - *Enterococcus* spp. (gastric surgery or pathology).
  - *Pseudomonas aeruginosa.*
  - **HACEK organisms**:
    - **H**: *Haemophilus aphrophilus*, *Haemophilus paraphrophilus* and *Haemophilus parainfluenzae*;
    - **A**: *Actinobacillus actinomycetemcomitans*;
    - **C**: *Cardiobacterium hominis*;
    - **E**: *Eikenella corrodens*;
    - **K**: *Kingella kingae.*
- **Fungi**:
  - *Candida* spp.;
  - *Aspergillus* spp.;
  - *Histoplasma* spp.

> **MICRO-facts**
>
> **Substances** added to **illicit drugs** to increase their weight (e.g. cement) cause **myocardial damage** and increase the risk of **endocarditis**.

## AETIOLOGY

- There are two main risk factors for infective endocarditis:
  - **Bacteraemia**:
    - IVDU;
    - dental treatment or poor oral hygiene;
    - infections (e.g. skin, urinary tract infection and respiratory);
    - cardiac surgery (e.g. pacemaker insertion);
    - venous procedures (e.g. cannula or central venous line).
  - **Abnormal cardiac epithelium**:
    - **Iatrogenic**: prosthetic heart valves.
    - **Heart valve disease**:
      - rheumatic fever;
      - mitral or aortic regurgitation.
    - **Structural defects**:
      - ventricular septal defect;
      - patent ductus arteriosus;
      - hypertrophic cardiomyopathy;
      - calcified aortic stenosis.
  - Structurally normal heart valves can also become infected, especially with *S. aureus* and *Streptococcus pneumoniae.*

## PATHOPHYSIOLOGY

- Structurally weakened and damaged endocardium (particularly valves and the chordae tendineae) is susceptible to colonization with an infective organism, especially if a thrombus (platelets and fibrin) has already been deposited.
- This process of infection and deposition of thrombus continues, forming the characteristic vegetation lesion.
- As the disease progresses, the valve is destroyed and regurgitation or obstruction develops.
- Thrombi from the vegetation can embolize to distant organs and impair their blood supply.
- In addition, infective organisms can enter the circulation and form immune complexes with systemic impact.

## SYMPTOMS

- **General**:
  - fever and night sweats;

  - malaise;
  - weight loss.
- **Cardiac**: heart failure.
- **Renal**: haematuria.
- **Bones and joints**: arthralgia.

> **MICRO-facts**
>
> All patients with a **fever** and **new** or **changing murmur** should be investigated for **infective endocarditis**.

## SIGNS

- **General**: clubbing.
- **Cardiac**: murmur (new or changed).
- **Spleen**: splenomegaly.
- **Immune complex deposition** (now less common as disease discovered earlier):
  - **Hands**:
    - **Osler's nodes**: painful, red, raised lesions on pulps of fingers (pathognomonic).
    - **Janeway lesions**: red, painless macules on palm (pathognomonic).
    - **Splinter haemorrhages**: small and straight, red lesions under the nails; can also be caused by trauma.
  - **Eyes**:
    - **Roth's spots**: red lesions with a central pale zone (seen with fundoscopy).
  - **Skin**: petechiae.

## COMPLICATIONS

- Determined by the side of the heart with the lesion.
- **Right-hand side** (associated with IVDU):
  - pulmonary embolism;
  - lung abscess.
- **Left-hand side**:
  - **Renal failure**: immune complex deposition (glomerulonephritis) or decreased renal blood flow.
  - **Stroke**: thrombotic embolism or cerebral haemorrhage.
  - **Distal gangrene**: fingers or toes owing to embolism or vasculitis.
  - **Gastrointestinal embolism**: thrombi can cause bowel ischaemia and infarction.
  - Splenic infarction.

## INVESTIGATIONS

- **Urine dipstick**: microscopic haematuria.
- **Blood tests**:
  - **Full blood count**: anaemia (normocytic normochromic) and neutrophil leucocytosis.
  - **Urea and electrolytes**: renal function.
  - **C-reactive protein (CRP) and erythrocyte sedimentation rate (ESR)**: raised.
- **Blood cultures**: three separate sets.
- **Echocardiography**:
  - transoesophageal (more sensitive) or transthoracic;
  - can reveal vegetations or valvular dysfunction.
- **Chest radiograph**: heart failure.

## DUKE'S CRITERIA

- Scoring scale used to diagnose infective endocarditis.
- **Method**: add up major and minor criteria.
- **Scores**:
  - **Definite infective endocarditis**: two major or one major and three minor or five minor.
  - **Possible**: one major and one minor or three minor.
- **Major criteria**:
  - **Positive blood culture**:
    - endocarditis-causing organism in two separate blood cultures;
    - persistently positive blood culture (e.g. samples more than 12 hours apart or all three positive).
  - **Endocardial involvement**:
    - positive echocardiogram visualization of intracardiac lesion;
    - new valvular regurgitation (change in pre-existing murmur does not count).
- **Minor criteria**:
  - **Fever**: greater than 38°C.
  - **Predisposing factors**: IVDU or pre-existent cardiac lesion.
  - Immunological/vascular signs.
  - **Positive blood culture/echocardiogram**: does not meet above criteria.

## MANAGEMENT

- **Medication**:
  - Consult with microbiologists and treat according to antibiotic sensitivities.
  - **Empirical**: flucloxacillin or benzylpenicillin and gentamicin.
  - **Empirical with cardiac prostheses**: vancomycin and rifampicin.

  - **Staphylococci**: flucloxacillin or vancomycin and rifampicin (penicillin allergy or meticillin-resistant *Staphylococcus aureus*).
  - **Streptococci**: benzylpenicillin or vancomycin (if penicillin allergic or resistance) and gentamicin.
  - **Enterococci**: amoxicillin or vancomycin (if penicillin allergic or resistance) and gentamicin.
  - **HACEK organisms**: amoxicillin or ceftriaxone (resistance) and gentamicin.
  - **Fungi**: choices include amphotericin, flucytosine and fluconazole (seek advice from microbiology).
- **Surgical**: prosthetic valves for significant valvular damage or infected prostheses.

### PREVENTION

- **Antibiotic prophylaxis**: the National Institute for Health and Clinical Excellence does not recommend offering antibiotic prophylaxis for patients with predisposing cardiac lesions undergoing procedures that could cause bacteraemia (e.g. dental work).

> **MICRO-reference**
>
> National Institute for Health and Clinical Excellence. *Prophylaxis against infective endocarditis*. Clinical Guidance 64. London, UK: NICE, 2008. Available from: www.guidance.nice.org.uk/CG64

## 9.2 RHEUMATIC FEVER

### DEFINITION

- A multisystem inflammatory reaction that follows group A β-haemolytic streptococcal infection.

### EPIDEMIOLOGY

- Most common in children and young adults.
- Rare in developed countries since the advent of antibiotic therapy and improved sanitation.
- Continues to be a common problem in Africa, southern America and the Middle East.

### INFECTIVE AGENTS

- Rheumatic fever occurs after pharyngeal infection with *Streptococcus pyogenes* (group A β-haemolytic streptococci).

## PATHOPHYSIOLOGY

- Rheumatic fever is an autoimmune response to *S. pyogenes* infection.
- The body forms antibodies to M proteins that are found on the cell wall of *S. pyogenes.*
- These antigens are structurally similar to natural connective tissues in the heart and joints (molecular mimicry). Accordingly, the anti-streptococcal antibodies cross-react with these tissues and cause inflammatory damage.

## REVISED DUCKETT JONES CRITERIA

- A scoring scale based on symptoms and signs that is used to diagnose rheumatic fever.
- **Method**: demonstrate recent streptococcal infection and then add up major and minor criteria.
- **Evidence of a recent streptococcal infection**:
  - history of scarlet fever;
  - elevated anti-streptolysin O titre (>200 U/mL; antibody to streptococcal haemolysin molecule);
  - other streptococcal antibodies such as DNase B or hyaluronidase;
  - positive throat cultures for streptococcal infection.
- **Major criteria**:
  - **Carditis**:
    - tachycardia;
    - murmur (new or changed);
    - pericardial rub;
    - elevated ST segments (pericarditis) or inverted/flattened T waves (myocarditis).
  - **Subcutaneous nodules**: small, painless, mobile and hard nodules over joints.
  - **Erythema marginatum**: erythematous, non-painful lesions on the trunk and peripheries that come and go.
  - **Arthritis**: polyarthritis, favouring large joints and short lasting.
  - **Sydenham's chorea (St Vitus' dance)**: rapid, jerky involuntary movements with a preceding change in mood and character.
- **Minor criteria**:
  - fever;
  - arthralgia (not counted if major criteria arthritis is present);
  - previous rheumatic fever;
  - raised ESR or CRP;
  - prolonged PR interval (not if major criteria carditis present);
  - leucocytosis.
- **Scores**:
  - **Definite rheumatic fever**: recent streptococcal infection and two major criteria or one major criterion and two minor criteria.

## COMPLICATIONS

- Chronic disease with recurring acute episodes will develop in up to 60% of patients and can present with valvular stenosis or regurgitation.
- These lesions may result in heart failure and increase the risk of infective endocarditis.

## INVESTIGATIONS

- **Throat swab**: culture to demonstrate recent or current streptococcal infection.
- **Blood tests**:
  - **ESR and CRP**: raised.
  - **Serological tests**: anti-streptolysin O titre and DNase B or hyaluronidase antibodies.
- **Electrocardiogram**: prolonged PR interval, elevated ST segments (pericarditis) or inverted/flattened T waves (myocarditis).
- **Echocardiogram**: valvular damage.

## MANAGEMENT

- **General**: bed rest until fever, arthritis or carditis has improved.
- **Medication**:
  - **Streptococcal infection**: phenoxymethylpenicillin.
  - **Analgesia**: high-dose aspirin, monitor salicylate level and be aware of tinnitus and metabolic acidosis caused by toxicity.
  - **Active carditis**: prednisolone.
  - **Chronic recurrence**: phenoxymethylpenicillin daily until 20 years old (infection is less common at this age).

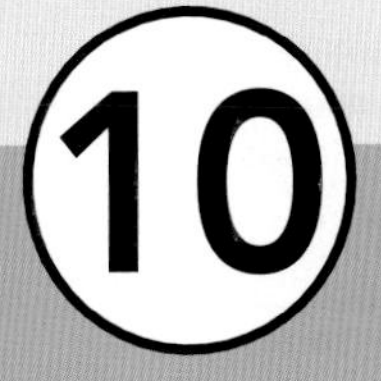

# 10 Haematological infections and HIV

## 10.1 MALARIA

### DEFINITION

- Malaria is an infection of red blood cells caused by a protozoan parasite.

### EPIDEMIOLOGY

- Endemic malaria is predominantly found in the tropics and subtropics.

### INFECTIVE AGENTS

- Protozoan parasite.
- Four different species relevant to man (malarial disease in brackets):
    - *Plasmodium falciparum* (malignant tertian malaria);
    - *Plasmodium vivax* (benign tertian malaria);
    - *Plasmodium ovale* (ovale tertian malaria);
    - *Plasmodium malariae* (quartan malaria);

> **MICRO-facts**
>
> **Tertian** (48 hours) and **quartan** (72 hours) refer to the **cyclical nature** of **malarial fever**, i.e. fever every 3 days.

### LIFE CYCLE

- Two phases with two hosts:
    - **Sexual**: *Anopheles* mosquito.
    - **Asexual**: vertebrate host (e.g. human).
- *Plasmodium* spp. has multiple forms throughout its life cycle.

#### Transmission

- *Plasmodium* spp. transmitted to human host via female *Anopheles* mosquito (blood meal required to produce eggs).
- Sporozoites present in mosquito salivary glands enter bloodstream when human is bitten.

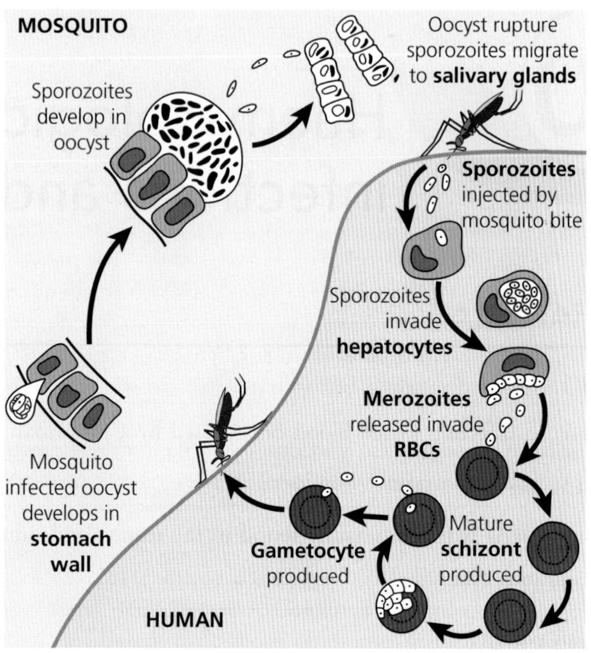


Fig. 10.1 *Plasmodium* spp. life cycle. RBC, red blood cell.

## Hepatic stage

- Sporozoites enter hepatocytes and either:
  - multiply and mature over 1–2 weeks (asymptomatic period) to form hepatic schizonts; *or*
  - form latent hepatic schizonts (hypnozoites) that reactivate (months to 5 years later) in 5–10% (*P. ovale* and *P. vivax* only).
- Hepatic schizonts subsequently rupture and release merozoites into the bloodstream.

## Erythrocytic stage

- Merozoites invade and replicate within red blood cells, forming erythrocytic schizonts.
- The erythrocytic schizont subsequently haemolyses and releases more merozoites into the bloodstream.
- This cycle of infection, multiplication and rupture repeats.

## Reproductive stage

- Some merozoites develop into gametocytes.
- *Plasmodium* spp. gametocytes re-enter the *Anopheles* mosquito when an infected individual is rebitten.

- *Plasmodium* spp. reproduction occurs in the gut of the mosquito.
- The new sporozoites progress to the salivary glands for transmission to a new host.

## IMMUNITY

- **Innate immunity**: some red blood cell defects (e.g. sickle cell disease, thalassaemia and glucose 6-phosphate dehydrogenase deficiency) are partially protective.
- **Acquired immunity**:
    - multiple previous malarial infections (immunity declines with pregnancy, severe illness and surgery);
    - neonates in endemic areas have approximately 6 months' immunity from maternal antibodies.

## SYMPTOMS

- **Incubation period**: 7–30 days (varies depending upon species).
- Flu-like prodromal phase in some cases.
- **Paroxysmal fever** (up to 10 hours):
    - Secondary to haemolysis of erythrocytic schizonts.
    - **Three phases**:
        - **Cold stage**: rigors.
        - **Hot stage**: pyrexia (may exceed 40°C), vomiting and convulsions.
        - **Sweating stage**: resolving fever, excess sweating and sleep.
    - Fever can be continuous or a subsequent asymptomatic phase can occur as further erythrocytic schizonts form:
        - ***P. ovale*** and ***P. vivax***: 48 hours (tertian).
        - ***P. falciparum***: less predictable.
        - ***P. malariae***: 72 hours (quartan).
- **Other symptoms**:
    - diarrhoea;
    - abdominal pain;
    - cough;
    - headache;

> **MICRO-facts**
>
> **Suspect malaria** in all patients with a **fever** and a recent **travel history**.

## SIGNS

- Anaemia and jaundice (secondary to haemolysis).
- Hepatosplenomegaly.
- Tachycardia.

- Flow murmur.
- Respiratory distress.

## COMPLICATIONS

- *P. malariae* infection can persist for many years, often asymptomatically.
- The majority of complications are due to *P. falciparum* infection in the non-immune.
- *P. falciparum* can cause red blood cell sequestration, which results in microcirculation disturbance.
- **Neurological**:
  - **Cerebral malaria**:
    - **Clinical features**: headache, altered consciousness, fits, focal neurological deficits, coma and death.
    - 20% mortality and 5% neurological sequelae.
- **Respiratory**: acute respiratory distress syndrome.
- **Haematological**:
  - disseminated intravascular coagulation;
  - severe anaemia.
- **Metabolic**:
  - hypoglycaemia;
  - metabolic acidosis.
- **Renal**:
  - renal failure (hypovolaemia can cause acute tubular necrosis);
  - blackwater fever (haemoglobinuria discolours the urine black).
- **Pregnancy**:
  - decreased natural immunity results in more severe disease;
  - increased risk of miscarriage, prematurity and low birth weight.

## INVESTIGATIONS

- **Thick and thin blood films**:
  - Gold standard investigation.
  - Three negative blood films required to exclude malaria.
  - **Thick blood film**: for general malaria diagnosis.
  - **Thin blood film**: to diagnose species of *Plasmodium*.
- Newer methods also available such as rapid antigen detection tests.

## MANAGEMENT

- Malaria must be treated as quickly as possible after the initial diagnosis.
- Benign uncomplicated malaria can be treated in an outpatient setting.
- **Anti-malarial chemotherapy**:

- Consider patient's travel history and the local *Plasmodium* resistance.
- ***P. falciparum***:
  - quinine and doxycycline or clindamycin;
  - atovaquone with proguanil (Malarone);
  - artemisinins (e.g. artemether with lumefantrine (Riamet)).
  - **Pregnancy**: quinine and clindamycin.
- ***P. malariae***: chloroquine.
- ***P. vivax*** and ***P. ovale***: chloroquine, then radical cure with primaquine to eliminate hypnozoites.

- **Anti-pyretic**:
  - paracetamol;
  - fanning and sponging.

## PREVENTION

- **General advice**:
  - cover exposed skin after dusk;
  - insecticide-treated mosquito nets (usually permethrin);
  - *N*, *N*-diethyl-meta-toluamide (DEET)-containing lotions and sprays.
- **Chemoprophylaxis** (dependent on local patterns of resistance):
  - **Chloroquine**: areas with low risk of chloroquine-resistant *P. falciparum*.
  - **Chloroquine with proguanil (Paludrine/Avloclor)**: low-risk areas, pregnancy and adverse effects with other anti-malarials.
  - **Mefloquine (Lariam)**: areas with chloroquine-resistant *P. falciparum*; weekly dose.
  - **Doxycycline**: areas with chloroquine or mefloquine resistance; daily dose.
  - **Proguanil hydrochloride with atovaquone (Malarone)**: high-risk areas; daily dose.

> **MICRO-facts**
>
> **Photosensitivity** develops in **15–20%** of people taking **doxycycline** – this can be a problem in **sunny malarious** countries.

# 10.2 HUMAN IMMUNODEFICIENCY VIRUS/ ACQUIRED IMMUNE DEFICIENCY SYNDROME

## EPIDEMIOLOGY

- Human immunodeficiency virus (HIV) was discovered in 1983.
- In 2008, the global prevalence of HIV was estimated to be 33.4 million.

- The greatest burden of disease is still in sub-Saharan Africa, but levels are rising in developed and non-developed countries alike.
- Two strains have been isolated (HIV-1 and HIV-2). HIV-2 is mainly prevalent in west Africa and has a slower disease progression than HIV-1.

## ROUTES OF TRANSMISSION

- **Sexual**:
  - heterosexual and homosexual intercourse;
  - anal intercourse poses the highest risk.
- **Vertical**:
  - blood transference *in utero*;
  - during labour;
  - breast milk.

> **MICRO-facts**
>
> The majority of **vertical transmission** occurs during **labour**. Appropriate **anti-retroviral** medication and **caesarean section** dramatically reduces the **risk**.

- **Blood products**: infected, non-screened blood used for transfusion.
- **Intravenous drug use**: sharing of infected needles and/or syringes.

## LIFE CYCLE

- HIV replication causes progressive destruction of T helper cells (CD4 cells).
- This results in a state of immunodeficiency through impaired cell-mediated immunity.
- Individuals are therefore more susceptible to infections and diseases that a healthy immune system would have been capable of clearing.

## STAGES OF INFECTION

- **Incubation**:
  - 2–4 weeks;
  - all tests will be negative.
- **Seroconversion illness**:
  - fever;
  - muscle aches;
  - lymphadenopathy;
  - maculopapular rash;
  - diarrhoea;
  - may be mistaken for infectious mononucleosis.

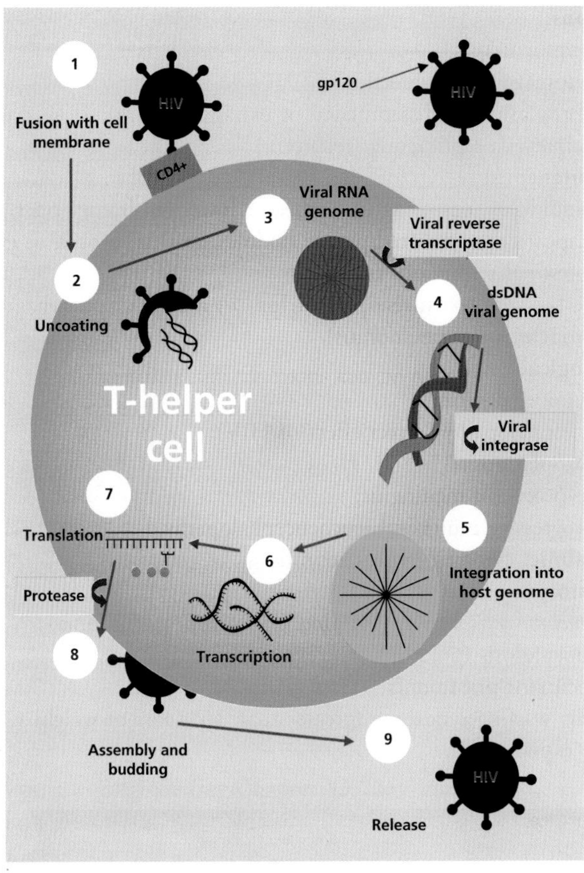


Fig. 10.2 Human immunodeficiency virus life cycle.

- **Latent period**: up to 10 years without any symptoms.
- **Disease progression**: development of acquired immune deficiency syndrome (AIDS). This is said to have occurred when the patient has either:
  - developed an AIDS-defining illness; *or*
  - has a CD4 count of $<200$ cells/μL.

## ACQUIRED IMMUNE DEFICIENCY SYNDROME-DEFINING ILLNESSES

- **Genitourinary**: invasive cervical carcinoma.
- **Gastrointestinal**: cryptosporidiosis (chronic for $>1$ month).
- **Haematology**:
  - Burkitt's lymphoma;
  - primary lymphoma of the brain.

- **Infections**:
  - cryptococcosis;
  - cytomegalovirus infection;
  - histoplasmosis (disseminated or extrapulmonary);
  - *Salmonella* septicaemia (recurrent).
- **Mucocutaneous**:
  - candidiasis (oesophagus, trachea or lower respiratory tract);
  - Kaposi's sarcoma (red/purple nodules on skin, mouth or gastro-intestinal/respiratory tract);
  - herpes simplex (ulcers present for >1 month or oesophagitis, bronchitis or pneumonitis).
- **Neurological**:
  - cytomegalovirus;
  - encephalopathy (direct effect of HIV);
  - toxoplasmosis;
  - cryptococcal meningitis;
  - progressive multifocal leucoencephalopathy.
- **Ophthalmic**: cytomegalovirus retinitis.
- **Respiratory**:
  - *Pneumocystis jiroveci* (*Pneumocystis carinii*) pneumonia;
  - tuberculosis (pulmonary or extrapulmonary);
  - recurrent pneumonia.
- **Systemic**: wasting syndrome (greater than 10% loss of weight without another explanation).

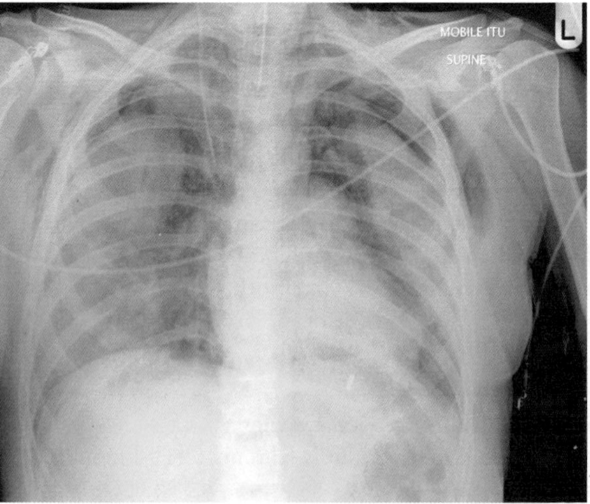


Fig. 10.3 Chest radiograph showing *Pneumocystis jiroveci* (*Pneumocystis carinii*) pneumonia infection. Courtesy of Dr I. Bickle, Northern General Hospital, Sheffield, UK.

## COMPLICATIONS

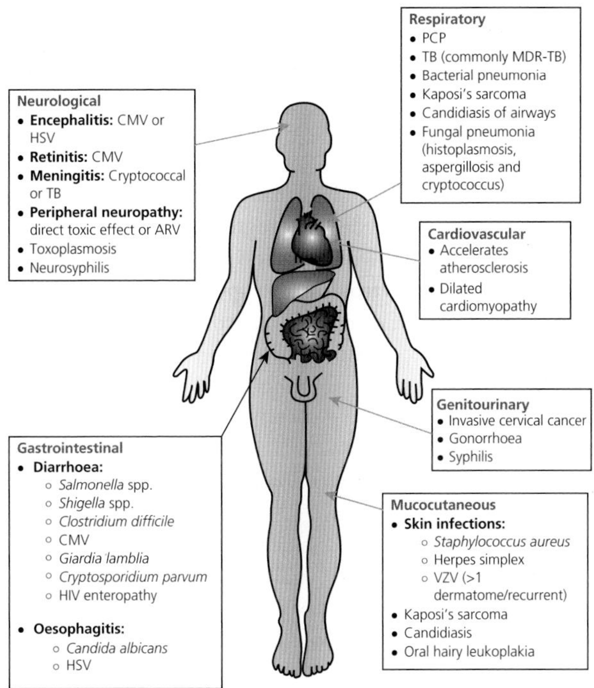


Fig. 10.4 Complications associated with human immunodeficiency syndrome/acquired immune deficiency syndrome. ARV, anti-retroviral; CMV, cytomegalovirus; HSV, herpes simplex virus; MDR-TB, multidrug-resistant TB; PCP, *Pneumocystis jiroveci* (*Pneumocystis carinii*) pneumonia; TB, tuberculosis; VZV, varicella zoster virus.

## DIAGNOSIS

- Antibody tests can be negative during the first few weeks post-infection. All patients should be positive 3 months after exposure and many will be by 6 weeks.
- **Initial test**: enzyme-linked immunosorbent assay (ELISA) technique to detect HIV-1 and HIV-2 antibodies and HIV-1 p24 antigen.
- **Confirmatory test**: if the ELISA test is positive, confirm infection and determine HIV strain by western blot.
- **Alternative techniques**:
  - polymerase chain reaction (PCR) for viral deoxyribonucleic acid (used to monitor treatment response and infection severity);
  - viral culture.

### MICRO-facts

**Human immunodeficiency virus** causes disease by **infection, tumour** or **direct toxic effect**.

## MANAGEMENT

- **Treatment**:
  - Treatment aims to reduce viral load and increase CD4 count. Both can be used as markers for disease progression.
  - Start treatment if CD4 count is less than 350 cells/mm$^3$.
  - **Highly active anti-retroviral therapy (HAART)**: combination of three main classes of drugs: (1) nucleoside reverse transcriptase inhibitors (NRTIs); (2) non-nucleoside reverse transcriptase inhibitors (NNRTIs); (3) protease inhibitors (PIs).
    - **Regimes**: two NRTIs + one NNRTI or one PI.
- **Ongoing management**:
  - monitor CD4 count and viral load (PCR) to assess disease progression and response to treatment;
  - regular clinic reviews to assess general health, opportunistic infections and side-effects of anti-retroviral therapy;
  - start co-trimoxazole prophylaxis against *Pneumocystis jiroveci* pneumonia if CD4 count less than 200 cells/mm$^3$.

### MICRO-facts

**Poor response** to **anti-microbials** is caused by:
non-compliance;
poor absorption (e.g. coeliac disease);
drug resistance.

### MICRO-reference

British HIV Association. ***British HIV Association guidelines for the treatment of HIV-1 infected adults with antiretroviral therapy 2008.*** London, UK: BHIVA, 2008. Available from: http//www.bhiva.org/documents/Guidelines/Treatment%20Guidelines/Current/TreatmentGuidelines2008.pdf

British HIV Association. ***UK national guidelines for HIV testing 2008.*** London, UK: BHIVA, 2008. Available from: http//www.bhiva.org/documents/Guidelines/Testing/GlinesHIVTest08.pdf

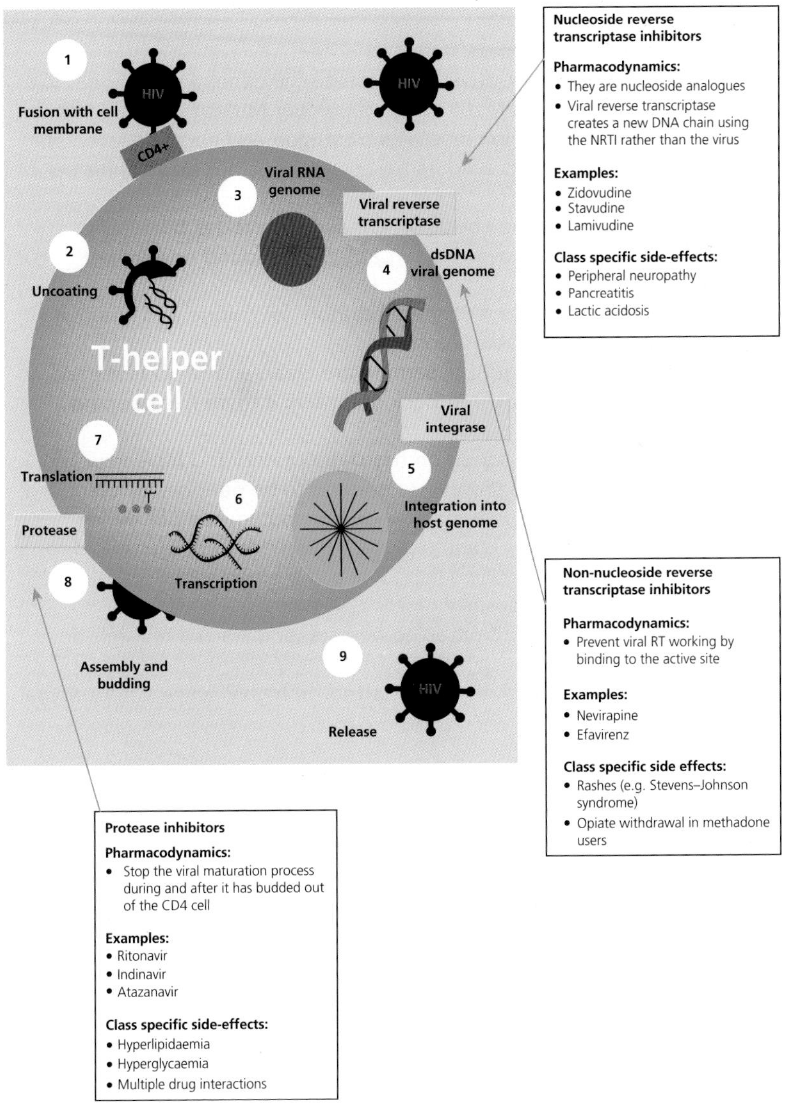


Fig. 10.5 Human immunodeficiency virus/acquired immune deficiency syndrome treatment: pharmacodynamics, examples and side-effects. NRTI, nucleoside reverse transcriptase inhibitor; RT, reverse transcriptase.

**MICRO-case**

Mr O, a 45 year old truck driver, presents to his general practitioner with increasing shortness of breath on exertion over the past 3 weeks with a non-productive cough. He complains of fatigue and episodic fever. He was previously well. He is a non-smoker with no other medical history of note.

On examination of the chest, Mr O has fine crackles bilaterally, tachycardia and tachypnoea. Nothing of note is found on general examination.

A sputum sample is sent to the laboratory for culture and Gram stain, and Mr O is sent for a radiograph.

The radiograph and sputum sample are clear, and Mr O is started on an antibiotic and told to come back in a week if there has been no improvement.

A week later, Mr O's condition has deteriorated and he is now very short of breath and looks unwell. He is found to be peripherally cyanosed.

He is sent to the hospital for an induced sputum sample, which confirms the presence of *Pneumocystis jiroveci*. Mr O is counselled for a human immunodeficiency virus (HIV) test and a blood sample is taken. He is confirmed to be HIV positive.

Mr O is immediately admitted to hospital and started on high-dose co-trimoxazole.

His $CD4^+$ count is 134, so he is started on highly active anti-retroviral therapy.

**Points to consider**:

- HIV should be considered in all patients presenting atypically.
- Generalized lymphadenopathy can be present even in asymptomatic patients with latent HIV infection.
- A detailed social and sexual history, if appropriate, can uncover major risk factors for acquiring HIV infection.

# 11 Genitourinary infections

## 11.1 URINARY TRACT INFECTION

### CYSTITIS

- **Epidemiology**:
  - extremely common in women owing to a short urethra and a high chance of contamination with perineal commensals;
  - should **always** be investigated in men (see below);
  - recurrent infection should **always** be investigated in children (see below).

> **MICRO-facts**
>
> **Bacterial colonization of long-term catheters is usual,** hence urine dipstick is almost always positive. Catheter urine samples should therefore not be sent unless the patient has clinical symptoms of a UTI.

- **Organisms**:
  - *Escherichia coli*;
  - *Proteus mirabilis*;
  - *Klebsiella pneumoniae*;
  - *Enterobacter*;
  - *Enterococcus* spp.;
  - *Staphylococcus saprophyticus*;
  - *Pseudomonas aeruginosa* (particularly from long-term catheters);
  - *Candida* spp. – may colonize catheters.
- **Risk factors**:
  - **Poor hygiene**:
    - females should be encouraged to wipe from urethra towards anus after using the toilet;
    - common in children and the elderly.
  - **Sexual activity in females**:
    - poor post-coital hygiene predisposes to urinary tract infection (UTI);

    - women are advised to pass urine immediately after intercourse to reduce the risk of infection.
  - **Structural**: due to outflow obstruction:
    - prostate – benign prostatic hypertrophy or malignancy;
    - vaginal prolapse in elderly women;
    - calculi;
    - strictures in the urethra;
    - bladder – tumours etc.
  - **Neurogenic** bladder, e.g. spinal cord lesion.
  - **Immunocompromised**:
    - chemotherapy;
    - immune suppression;
    - diabetes mellitus.
  - Pregnancy.
  - Urethral catheters.
  - Tuberculosis.
  - Schistosomiasis.
- **Clinical features**:
  - increased frequency;
  - dysuria;
  - lower abdominal pain;
  - occasionally haematuria;
  - systemic illness e.g. pyrexia;
  - confusion, including delirium especially in the elderly.
- **Diagnosis**:
  - urine dipstick – positive for leukocytes, nitrites ± blood;
  - mid-stream urine for microscopy, culture and sensitivity (MC&S);
  - further investigation if in men, or recurrent especially in children, e.g. prostate-specific antigen, prostate examination, etc.
- **Treatment**:
  - trimethoprim, nitrofurantoin, co-amoxiclav, cephalexin;
  - for treatment of tuberculosis or schistosomiasis see Chapter 7, Respiratory infections or Chapter 5, Helminths.

## PYELONEPHRITIS

- **Epidemiology**: common.
- **Organisms**:
  - *E. coli*;
  - *P. mirabilis*;
  - *K. pneumoniae*;
  - *Enterobacter*;
  - *Enterococcus* spp.;
  - *S. saprophyticus*;

  - *P. aeruginosa* (particularly from long-term catheters);
  - *Candida* spp. – may colonize catheters.
  - Other, e.g. from haematogenous spread of distal infection.
- **Risk factors**: as for cystitis but also:
  - **Structural problems**:
    - **Vesicoureteric reflux**:
      - due to incompetent valves between bladder and ureters;
      - common in children; often resolves with age, but may require surgery.
    - **Outflow obstruction**:
      - anything which blocks passage of urine through the tract;
      - prostate – benign prostatic hypertrophy or malignancy;
      - bladder – tumours, etc.;
      - ureters – strictures, stones, malignancy, retroperitoneal fibrosis;
      - kidneys – malignancy, stones, etc.
  - Urethral catheters or cystoscopy.
  - Systemic sepsis with haematogenous spread to kidneys.
- **Clinical features**:
  - abdominal pain – loin pain;
  - systemic sepsis, rigors and pyrexia;
  - pyuria;
  - haematuria.
- **Diagnosis**:
  - urine dipstick – positive for leucocytes, nitrites $\pm$ blood;
  - mid-stream urine for MC&S;
  - renal ultrasound to exclude hydronephrosis;
  - clinical differentiation from cystitis – if systemic sepsis or loin pain present, assume pyelonephritis.
- **Treatment**: gentamicin or co-amoxiclav.

## 11.2 CANDIDIASIS (THRUSH)

- **Organism**: *Candida albicans.*
- **Epidemiology**: up to 20% of women will suffer from thrush in their lifetime.
- **Risk factors**:
  - pregnancy;
  - diabetes mellitus;
  - immunocompromised states;
  - antibiotic use.
- **Clinical features**:
  - pruritus;
  - cottage cheese or curdy discharge;

- vulval irritation;
- superficial dyspareunia;
- dysuria;
- reddened vagina and vulva.
- **Diagnosis**:
  - **Vaginal wall swab**:
    - **Culture**: Gram-positive spores.
    - **Microscopy**: spores and pseudohyphae.
- **Treatment**: clotrimazole (pessary or cream) or fluconazole.

## 11.3 BACTERIAL VAGINOSIS

- **Organism**:
  - Overgrowth of normal vaginal flora with anaerobes:
    - *Gardnerella vaginalis*;
    - *Mycoplasma hominis*;
    - *Bacteroides* spp.
- **Epidemiology**: 12% of women will develop bacterial vaginosis in their lifetime.
- **Clinical features**:
  - grey-white discharge with a fishy odour;
  - up to 50% asymptomatic;
  - increased risk of premature labour.
- **Diagnosis**:
  - **Amsel criteria** (at least three for diagnosis):
    - **Discharge**: grey-white with fishy odour.
    - **pH**: increased vaginal pH (>4.5).
    - **Whiff test**: 10% potassium hydroxide mixed with vaginal discharge produces a fishy odour.
    - **Clue cells**: vaginal squamous epithelial cells coated with bacteria seen on microscopy.
- **Treatment**: metronidazole or clindamycin (topical).

## 11.4 CHLAMYDIA

- **Organism**: *Chlamydia trachomatis* (serotypes D–K).
- **Epidemiology**: 5% sexually active women.
- **Sites of infection**:
  - **Women**: endocervix, urethra, pharynx and rectum.
  - **Men**: urethra, pharynx and rectum.
- **Clinical features**:
  - **Women**:
    - asymptomatic;

> **MICRO-facts**
>
> Up to **80%** of **women** and **50%** of **men** can be **asymptomatic** during **chlamydia** infection.

    - vaginal discharge;
    - post-coital or inter-menstrual bleeding;
    - lower abdominal pain.
  - **Men**:
    - Asymptomatic.
    - **Urethritis**:
      - clear and scanty urethral discharge;
      - dysuria.
  - **Neonates**: ophthalmia neonatorum.
- **Complications**:
  - **Women**:
    - pelvic inflammatory disease (tubal damage can cause infertility);
    - Reiter's syndrome (triad of conjunctivitis, reactive arthritis and urethritis).
  - **Men**:
    - epididymo-orchitis;
    - prostatitis (with rectal infection);
    - proctitis;
    - Reiter's syndrome.
- **Diagnosis**:
  - *C. trachomatis* is an obligate intracellular bacterium that is difficult to culture. Accordingly, enzyme-linked immunosorbent assay or immunofluorescence testing of patient samples is the favoured diagnostic option.
  - **Women**: endocervical or urethral swab.
  - **Men**:
    - urine (first-voided urine);
    - urethral swab.
- **Treatment**: doxycycline or azithromycin or erythromycin.

> **MICRO-facts**
>
> Up to **50%** of **women** and **10%** of **men** can be **asymptomatic** during **gonorrhoeal** infection.

## 11.5 GONORRHOEA

- **Organism**: *Neisseria gonorrhoeae.*
- **Epidemiology**: commonly found with chlamydia infections.
- **Sites of infection**: mucosal epithelium (e.g. urethra, rectum, cervix, conjunctiva and oropharynx).
- **Clinical features**:
  - **Women**:
    - asymptomatic;
    - vaginal discharge;
    - pelvic pain;
    - irregular vaginal bleeding;
    - dysuria.
  - **Men**:
    - asymptomatic;
    - purulent urethral discharge;
    - dysuria;
    - proctitis.
  - **Neonates**: ophthalmia neonatorum.
- **Complications**:
  - **Women**:
    - **Bartholin's abscess**: infection of the Bartholin's glands.
    - **Rectal infection**: local spread of vaginal infection.
    - **Fitz-Hugh–Curtis syndrome**: ascending infection causes a peri-hepatitis.
    - Pelvic inflammatory disease (tubal damage can cause infertility).
  - **Men**:
    - epididymo-orchitis;
    - prostatitis (with rectal infection).
  - **Both**:
    - septic arthritis (usually monoarticular);
    - reactive arthritis.
- **Diagnosis**:
  - **Microscopy**:
    - **Swab sites**: urethral, rectal, conjunctival.
    - Gram stain will show Gram-negative diplococci within neutrophils.
- **Treatment**: cefixime or ciprofloxacin.

**MICRO-facts**

**Chlamydia** and **gonorrhoea** can appear very similar clinically; however, the **urethral discharge** of men may give a clue:

**Chlamydia**: clear and scanty.

**Gonorrhoea**: purulent.

## 11.6 GENITAL WARTS

**MICRO-print**

Human papillomavirus 16 and 18 are oncogenic as they produce E6 and E7 proteins that inhibit tumour suppressor proteins:
**E6**: inhibits **p53**.
**E7**: inhibits retinoblastoma protein.

- **Organism**: human papillomavirus (HPV).
- **Epidemiology**: very common and highly infectious.
- **Clinical features**:
  - **Genital warts**:
    - **Women**: peri-anal region, vulva and perineum.
    - **Men**: penile shaft and meatus.
- **Complications**:
  - **Women**: HPV types 16 and 18 are linked to cervical intraepithelial neoplasia and therefore an increased risk of cervical cancer.
- **Diagnosis**: clinical.
- **Treatment**:
  - **Keratinized**: imiquimod cream or cryotherapy or electrocautery.
  - **Non-keratinized**: trichloroacetic acid or cryotherapy or podophyllin (topical) or imiquimod cream.
  - **Immunization (UK schedule)**: girls aged 12–13 years old, protects against HPV types 16 and 18.

## 11.7 GENITAL HERPES

- **Organism**: herpes simplex virus (commonly type 2 but also type 1).
- **Epidemiology**: common in 16–24 year olds.

- **Clinical features**:
  - **Genital herpes**:
    - **Ulcers**: painful and shallow on the infected site (e.g. genitals, rectum, mouth and oropharynx).
    - Lymphadenopathy.
    - Dysuria.
    - **Systemic symptoms**: fever, myalgia and headache.
- **Diagnosis**:
  - clinical;
  - swabs (from base of lesions for polymerase chain reaction).
- **Treatment**:
  - **Primary**: saltwater bathing or aciclovir or famciclovir or valaciclovir.
  - **Frequent recurrent attacks**: aciclovir or valaciclovir.

## 11.8 SYPHILIS

- **Organism**: *Treponema pallidum.*
- **Clinical features**:
  - **Primary syphilis**:
    - chancre (hard papule that ulcerates at infection site 10–90 days post-infection);
    - lymphadenopathy.
  - **Secondary syphilis** (4–10 weeks post chancre):
    - highly infectious papular rash (mucous membranes and skin, including soles and palms);
    - condylomata lata (wart-like lesions common in the peri-anal region);
    - generalized lymphadenopathy;
    - mucosal ulceration (mouth and genitals);
    - fever;
    - malaise;
    - arthralgia.
  - **Tertiary syphilis** (up to 50 years later):
    - Gummas (granulomatous lesions in the bones and viscera).
    - Ascending aortic aneurysm.
    - Aortic regurgitation (owing to aortic root dilatation).
    - **Neurosyphilis**:
      - meningitis;
      - cranial nerve palsies;
      - Argyll Robertson pupil (accommodation without reaction);

        - tabes dorsalis (demyelination in the dorsal roots);
        - generalized paralysis of the insane (dementia and weakness).
    - **Congenital syphilis**:
        - stillbirth;
        - failure to thrive.
- **Diagnosis**:
    - *T. pallidum* is difficult to culture; therefore, microscopy or serological tests are required.
    - Dark ground microscopy.
    - **Serological**: multiple tests are available and can be grouped as specific (treponemal) or non-specific (non-treponemal) (see Chapter 1, Bacteria).
- **Treatment**: benzathine benzylpenicillin or doxycycline or erythromycin.

Table 11.1 Non-specific and specific serological tests for diagnosing syphilis

| | NON-SPECIFIC (NON-TREPONEMAL) | SPECIFIC (TREPONEMAL) |
|---|---|---|
| Examples | VDRL<br>RPR | ELISA<br>FTA-ABS<br>TPHA<br>TPPA |
| Function | Screening (confirm positive result with specific test)<br>Monitor treatment response | Confirm positive non-specific test<br>Detecting early disease (less than 4 weeks post infection) |
| False positives | Leprosy<br>Malaria<br>Viral illness<br>Pregnancy<br>SLE | Other treponemal diseases (e.g. yaws, bejel or pinta)<br>*Borrelia* spp. infection<br>*Leptospira* spp. infection<br>Pregnancy<br>Diabetes mellitus |

ELISA, enzyme-linked immunosorbent assay; FTA-ABS, fluorescent treponemal antibody absorption; RPR, rapid plasma reagent; SLE systemic lupus erythematosus; TPHA, *Treponema pallidum* haemagglutination assay; TPPA, *Treponema pallidum* particle agglutination; VDRL, Venereal Disease Research Laboratory.

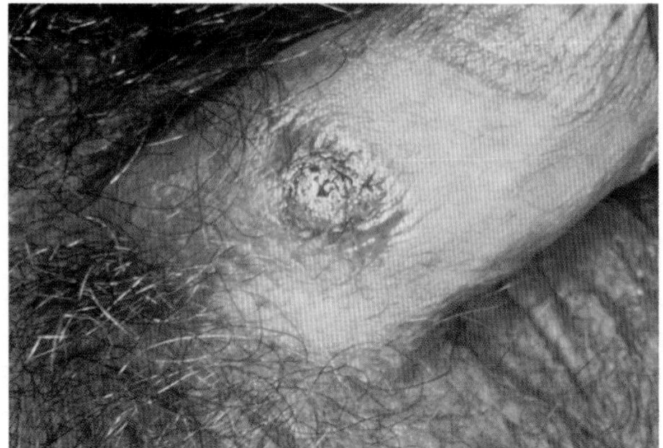

Fig. 11.1 Primary chancre at the base of a penis. Courtesy of the US Centers of Disease Control and Prevention/Dr Gavin Hart and Dr N.J. Fiumara.

## 11.9 TRICHOMONIASIS

- **Organism**: *Trichomonas vaginalis.*
- **Epidemiology**: rare in the UK.
- **Clinical features**:
  - **Women**:
    - offensive and frothy grey-green vaginal discharge;
    - vulval irritation;
    - dyspareunia;
    - multiple haemorrhages on cervix (strawberry cervix).
  - **Men**:
    - dysuria;
    - increased urinary frequency;
    - urethral discharge.
- **Diagnosis**: dark ground microscopy of vaginal discharge.
- **Treatment**: metronidazole.

> **MICRO-facts**
>
> **Men** commonly present as the **asymptomatic** partner of an infected female – **both** should be **treated** to avoid reinfection.
> *Trichomonas vaginalis* are flagellated protozoa, so can be seen 'swimming' when viewed under the microscope.

## 11.10 TOXIC SHOCK SYNDROME

- **Organism**: *Staphylococcus aureus.*
- **Risk factors**:
  - tampon use (frequency has fallen with newer tampons);
  - infected intrauterine contraceptive device;
  - surgical wound infection.
- **Pathology**:
  - *S. aureus* produces a supertoxin called toxic shock syndrome toxin (TSST-1).
  - This toxin is able to activate T cells via major histocompatibility complex II binding without antigen processing by antigen-presenting cells.
  - This mass activation of T cells results in a cytokine storm and subsequently shock.
- **Clinical features**:
  - Shock (hypotension and tachycardia).
  - Fever.
  - Diffuse macular rash.
  - **Multi-organ involvement**: renal failure, altered conscious level, abnormal liver function tests and vomiting or diarrhoea.
- **Diagnosis**: clinical.
- **Treatment**: flucloxacillin.

### MICRO-reference

National Institute of Health and Clinical Excellence. *Prevention of sexually transmitted infections and under 18 conceptions.* London, UK: NICE, 2007. Available from: http://guidance.nice.org.uk/PH3

### MICRO-case

Mr P, a 27 year old office worker, presents to the genitourinary medicine clinic with urethral discharge and pain on urination. On questioning about his sexual history, he reports to have abstained from sex since ending his relationship with his partner after she admitted infidelity.

On examination of the genitalia there is purulent urethral discharge but no other abnormalities. On general examination he is found to have reddened eyes, which he reports have been dry and sore. On further questioning, he says that his left knee has been swollen and painful. The knee is visibly swollen and a patellar tap confirms the presence of an effusion.

*continued...*

*continued...*

A urethral swab is taken. This shows obligate intracellular organisms – *Chlamydia trachomatis*.

Mr P is given a stat dose of azithromycin for the chlamydia infection, non-steroidal anti-inflammatory drugs for his knee pain and lubricating eye drops for the conjunctivitis. Contacts of Mr P are traced and tested.

Mr P makes a full recovery.

**Points to note**:

- Reiter's disease (classical triad of conjunctivitis, urethritis and arthritis) is associated with chlamydia infection.
- Chlamydia and gonorrhoea infection are very difficult to distinguish clinically. Disseminated gonococcal infection can also cause arthritis, but Reiter's disease is much more likely to be caused by chlamydia.
- Reactive arthritis usually settles and completely resolves, but a relapsing and remitting form of the disease can remain, which would need to be treated with disease-modifying anti-rheumatic drugs or steroids.
- Contact tracing is very important in the treatment of sexually transmitted infections.
- Chlamydia is commonly asymptomatic in both men and women.

# 12 Nervous system infections

## 12.1 MENINGITIS AND ENCEPHALITIS

### DEFINITIONS

- **Meningitis**: inflammation of the meningeal membranes that surround the brain.
- **Encephalitis**: inflammation within the substance of the central nervous system.

### EPIDEMIOLOGY

- **Meningitis**: most common in children, particularly within the first 5 years of life.

### INFECTIVE AGENTS

- **Meningitis** can be caused by bacteria, viruses (most common) or fungi.
  - **Viral pathogens**: enteroviruses (Coxsackievirus, poliovirus and *Enterovirus*), varicella zoster virus (VZV) and herpes simplex virus (HSV) (types 1 and 2).
  - **Bacterial pathogens**: vary by age (see Fig. 6.1).

Table 12.1 Bacterial causes of meningitis by age group

| AGE | PATHOGEN |
|---|---|
| <1 month | • Group B *Streptococcus*<br>• *Escherichia coli*<br>• *Listeria monocytogenes* |
| 1 month to 15 years | • *Streptococcus pneumoniae*<br>• *Neisseria meningitidis*<br>• *Haemophilus influenzae* (type b) |
| Adults (>15 years) | • *Streptococcus pneumoniae*<br>• *Neisseria meningitidis* |
| Older Adults (>55 years) | • *Streptococcus pneumoniae*<br>• *Neisseria meningitidis*<br>• *Listeria monocytogenes* |

- **Encephalitis** is most commonly due to HSV-1 or -2, measles, mumps or may also be caused by Japanese B encephalitis (an arbovirus).

> **MICRO-facts**
>
> ***Haemophilus influenzae* (type b)** remains an important cause of **meningitis** in countries **without** a **vaccination programme**.

## SYMPTOMS

- Headache.
- Photophobia.
- Fever.
- Neck stiffness.
- Poor feeding or generally unhappy (young children).
- Altered consciousness or confusion: **consider encephalitis.**

## SIGNS

- Neck stiffness.
- Kernig's sign (extension of a flexed knee causes pain and resistance to movement).
- Brudzinski's sign (passive neck flexion causes bilateral hip and knee flexion).
- Bulging fontanelle (infants).

> **MICRO-facts**
>
> **Meningitis** and **meningococcal septicaemia** are **not** the same thing:
>
> **Meningococcal septicaemia**: meningococcal **purpura** and **sepsis**. Meningitis **may** also be present.
>
> **Meningitis**: headache, photophobia and fever.

## INVESTIGATIONS

- **Lumbar puncture (LP)**:
  - **Contraindications**: signs of raised intracranial pressure, focal neurological signs or respiratory distress.
  - **Tests**:
    - White cell count (with differential), protein, glucose.
    - Microscopy, culture and sensitivity.
    - **Polymerase chain reaction (PCR)**: enteroviruses, HSV (types 1 and 2), VZV, meningococcus and pneumococcus.
    - **Serum glucose**: if cerebral spinal fluid (CSF) glucose $<40\%$ serum glucose, this suggests bacterial meningitis.

- In practice, a LP is rarely performed in patients with systemic sepsis as the risk of introducing infection into the CSF and beyond outweighs the benefits. Accordingly, treatment is started empirically and a LP may be performed after clinical improvement.

Table 12.2 Characteristic changes in cerebral spinal fluid during meningitis

| | VIRAL | BACTERIAL | TUBERCULOSIS |
|---|---|---|---|
| White Cell Count | ↑Lymphocytes | ↑Polymorphs | ↑Lymphocytes |
| Glucose | Normal/↓ | ↓↓ | ↓↓↓ |
| Protein | Normal/↑ | ↑↑ | ↑↑↑ |

- **Septic screen**: especially blood cultures, throat swab and urine and stool samples.
- **CT scan**: brain (rule out raised intracranial pressure prior to LP and encephalitis).
- **Electroencephalogram**: may show typical changes of HSV encephalitis.

## MANAGEMENT

- **Community**: benzylpenicillin and arrange emergency transfer to hospital.
- **Hospital**:
  - **Empirical**: cefotaxime or ceftriaxone (in most cases the causative organism is not known when antibiotics are started).
  - **Meningococcus**: cefotaxime or benzylpenicillin or chloramphenicol (immediate hypersensitivity to penicillin or cephalosporins).
  - **Pneumococcus**: cefotaxime or benzylpenicillin.
  - ***H. influenzae***: cefotaxime.
  - ***Listeria monocytogenes***: amoxicillin and gentamicin.
  - **HSV meningitis or encephalitis**: intravenous aciclovir.
- **Close contact prophylaxis**:
  - **Meningococcus**: rifampicin or ciprofloxacin.
  - ***H. influenzae***: rifampicin.

### MICRO-facts

**Rapid antibiotic** treatment is **vital** but will **impair cultures**.

## COMPLICATIONS

- Hearing loss.
- Subdural effusion.
- Cerebral infarction.
- Hydrocephalus.

## MICRO-facts

A recent **Cochrane review** has shown that starting **dexamethasone** with **antibiotics** reduces **complications** associated with **bacterial meningitis**; however, this issue remains controversial.

## MICRO-reference

Brouwer MC, McIntyre P, de Gans J, *et al.* Corticosteroids for acute bacterial meningitis. *Cochrane Database of Systematic Reviews* 2010, Issue 9. Art. No.: **CD004405**. DOI: 10.1002/14651858.CD004405.pub3

## MICRO-case

Baby Matthew is a preterm infant (born at 28 weeks) and is 4 hours old. The nurses on the neonatal ward alert the junior doctor that he is unwell and has a high temperature.

On examination, he is floppy and unresponsive, with a temperature of 39°C. He also appears jaundiced.

Meningitis is suspected and intravenous (IV) cefotaxime and IV aciclovir are given immediately. Bloods are taken for a full blood count, urea and electrolytes, liver function tests and cultures. A urine sample is sent; a lumbar puncture performed; and a chest radiograph requested.

The lumbar puncture appeared cloudy, with increased polymorphs and protein and reduced glucose. The blood culture came back negative and the urine sample and radiograph showed no evidence of infection.

Baby Matthew remained on the neonatal intensive care unit for several weeks, but recovered. He was, however, found to be profoundly deaf as a result of his meningitis.

**Points to note**:

- Preterm infants are at a greatly increased risk of sepsis.
- Presentation of sepsis in neonates is non-specific and cultures should be taken from as many sites as possible to confirm a diagnosis.
- Blood cultures are often negative when taken after administration of antibiotics and should not be solely relied upon.
- Common organisms in neonates are bacteria that can colonize the birth canal and are picked up during labour. These include group B *Streptococcus, Listeria monocytogenes* and *Escherichia coli.*
- Viral polymerase chain reaction (PCR) for herpes simplex virus, varicella zoster virus and enteroviruses along with meningococcal and pneumococcal PCR are performed routinely on cerebrospinal fluid samples.

*continued...*

*continued...*

- Penicillin or a third-generation cephalosporin should be administered as soon as there is a suspicion of meningitis; a definitive diagnosis must not be waited for.
- There are many possible complications for children who survive meningitis, of which hearing loss and neurodevelopmental delay are two examples.

## 12.2 BOTULISM

### DEFINITION

- A flaccid paralysis caused by botulinum toxin production.

### INFECTIVE AGENTS

- *Clostridium botulinum.*

### PATHOPHYSIOLOGY

- *C. botulinum* spores contaminate soil and foodstuffs and can germinate and produce toxins in anaerobic environments (e.g. poorly sterilized canned food).
- *C. botulinum* produces a neurotoxin that prevents acetylcholine binding with the terminal membrane of neurones.
- This prevents the propagation of the action potential and subsequently muscle contraction cannot occur.

### CLINICAL FEATURES

- **Four Ds**:
  - **D**iplopia.
  - **D**ysphagia.
  - **D**ysarthria.
  - **D**ysphonia.
- Abdominal pain and diarrhoea.
- Paralysis begins in the head and travels downwards.
- Respiratory paralysis can be fatal.

### INVESTIGATIONS

- Clinical diagnosis.
- Detection of botulinum toxin in recently consumed food or faeces.

### MANAGEMENT

- **General**: ventilatory support.

- **Medication**: anti-toxin.

## 12.3 TETANUS

### DEFINITION

- Tetanus is caused by a toxin (tetanospasmin) that causes muscle spasms and painful contractions.

### INFECTIVE AGENTS

- *Clostridium tetani.*

### PATHOPHYSIOLOGY

- Following inoculation with *C. tetani* spores, tetanospasmin toxin is produced.
- Tetanospasmin blocks inhibitory neurones in the central nervous system, which results in sustained muscle contraction.

### CLINICAL FEATURES

- Painful muscle spasms (induced by noise or movement).
- Lockjaw (trismus).
- Risus sardonicus (hypertonic facial muscles produce a grin-like expression).
- Opisthotonus (arching of the body and neck extension due to spasm).
- Autonomic dysfunction (e.g. unstable blood pressure and arrhythmias).

### INVESTIGATIONS

- Clinical diagnosis.

### MANAGEMENT

- **General**: ventilatory support.
- **Medication**:
  - human tetanus immunoglobulin;
  - metronidazole or benzylpenicillin;
  - diazepam (relieves spasms).

## 12.4 POLIOMYELITIS

### DEFINITION

- Poliomyelitis is a viral infection characterized by flaccid paralysis.

### INFECTIVE AGENTS

- Poliovirus.

## PATHOPHYSIOLOGY

- Following ingestion, the poliovirus replicates and causes destruction of anterior (motor) horn cells and the motor cortex of the brain.
- Subsequently, the lower motor neurones degenerate and paralysis develops.
- Non-paralytic polio can occur.

## CLINICAL FEATURES

- **Asymptomatic infection**: over 90% of people infected with the poliovirus do not develop any disease.
- **Abortive poliomyelitis**: occurs in 4–5% of infections with myalgia, fever and sore throat.
- **Paralytic poliomyelitis** (less than 1%):
  - **Prodrome**: fever and myalgia.
  - **Paralysis**:
    - asymmetrical flaccid paralysis;
    - respiratory muscle weakness and airway collapse (bulbar palsy) can be fatal.
- **Non-paralytic poliomyelitis**: viral meningitis.
- **Post-polio syndrome**: fatigue and muscle weakness many years after an initial polio infection.

## INVESTIGATIONS

- PCR testing for viral ribonucleic acid or cell culture from CSF, faeces or throat swabs.
- CSF lymphocytosis.

## MANAGEMENT

- **General**:
  - bed rest;
  - ventilatory support if needed;
  - early physiotherapy may restore muscle power.
- **Prevention**: vaccine.

# 13 Skin infections

## 13.1 MOLLUSCUM CONTAGIOSUM

### DEFINITION

- Highly contagious viral skin infection causing wart-like lesions.

### EPIDEMIOLOGY

- Common worldwide.
- Typically affects children and young adults.

### INFECTIVE AGENTS

- A poxvirus (molluscum contagiosum virus).

### TRANSMISSION

- Direct contact with infected skin.

### CLINICAL FEATURES

- Pearly flesh-coloured lesions, typically in groups on face and genitalia.

### INVESTIGATIONS

- Clinical diagnosis.

### MANAGEMENT

- Lesions can be removed by cryotherapy or topical astringent agents such as potassium hydroxide.

## 13.2 FOLLICULITIS

### DEFINITION

- Inflammation of hair follicles.

## EPIDEMIOLOGY

- Typically affects children.

## INFECTIVE AGENTS

- *Staphylococcus aureus.*
- *Pseudomonas aeruginosa* (associated with new hot tubs).

## TRANSMISSION

- Follicles are initially damaged (e.g. shaving, tight-fitting clothing) and then later infected.

## CLINICAL FEATURES

- Erythematous pustules around the hair follicles.
- Pruritus.

## INVESTIGATIONS

- Clinical diagnosis.

## MANAGEMENT

- Antibiotics rarely used.
- Encourage skin cleansing.

# 13.3 FURUNCLE (BOIL) AND CARBUNCLE

## DEFINITION

- **Furuncle (boil)**: deeper infection of the hair follicle, extending to the dermis and subcutaneous tissue.
- **Carbuncle**: the convergence of several furuncles into a single lesion with multiple openings.

## INFECTIVE AGENTS

- *S. aureus.*
- Coliforms and anaerobes (peri-anal lesions).

## CLINICAL FEATURES

- **Furuncle**: erythematous, tender nodule.
- **Carbuncle**: multiple lesions with systemic symptoms (e.g. fever).

## INVESTIGATIONS

- Pus swab for microscopy, culture and sensitivity (MC&S).

### MANAGEMENT

- **Peri-anal abscess**: surgical excision and drainage.

### COMPLICATIONS

- Systemic infection.
- Bacteraemia.

## 13.4 IMPETIGO

### DEFINITION

- Superficial skin infection usually affecting the face.

### EPIDEMIOLOGY

- Spreads quickly among school children owing to close contact.

### RISK FACTORS

- Eczema.
- Skin wound.

### INFECTIVE AGENTS

- *S. aureus* (most common).
- *Streptococcus pyogenes.*

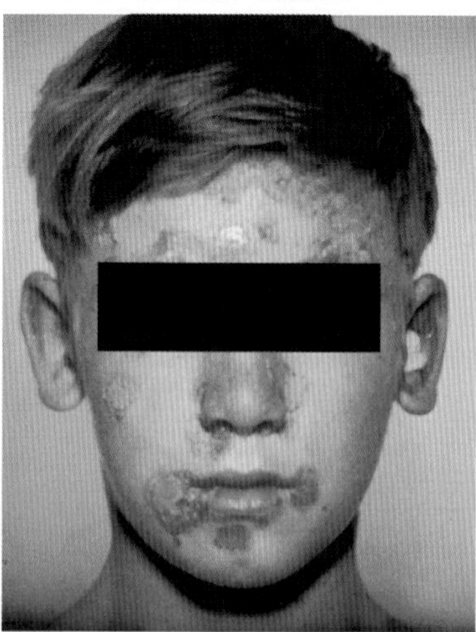

Fig. 13.1 Impetigo affecting the face. Courtesy of the Academic Department of Infection & Immunity, University of Sheffield, UK.

### TRANSMISSION

- Direct skin-to-skin contact.

### CLINICAL FEATURES

- Initially vesicles (typically around the mouth) that later burst and form the characteristic yellow scabs.

### INVESTIGATIONS

- Clinical diagnosis.
- Nasal swab to detect staphylococci colonization.

### MANAGEMENT

- Oral flucloxacillin and clearance of nasal staphylococci colonization.

## 13.5 ERYSIPELAS AND CELLULITIS

### DEFINITION

- **Cellulitis**: infection of the lower epidermis, dermis and subcutaneous tissues.
- **Erysipelas**: infection of the dermis caused by group A streptococci ('streptococcal cellulitis').

### RISK FACTORS

- Minor skin wound (e.g. burns, insect bites, cracked skin and cannula insertion site).
- Dermatitis.
- Peripheral vascular disease.

### INFECTIVE AGENTS

- **Cellulitis**:
  - *S. aureus*, including methicillin-resistant *S. aureus* (MRSA);
  - *S. pyogenes*;
  - Coliforms (immobile patients);
  - *P. aeruginosa*.
- **Erysipelas**: *S. pyogenes*.

> **MICRO-facts**
>
> **Coliforms** and ***Pseudomonas aeruginosa*** commonly cause **cellulitis** in **immobile** patients.
>
> *continued...*

*continued...*

***Staphylococcus aureus*** and ***Streptococcus pyogenes*** are common skin commensals. Once they break the outer skin barrier, they may become pathogenic, affecting the dermis, lower epidermis or subcutaneous tissues.

## TRANSMISSION

- Infection by normal skin flora.
- Direct contact with wounded skin.

## CLINICAL FEATURES

- **Cellulitis**: erythematous (indistinct margins), swollen and painful lesion that spreads. Typically on the limbs.
- **Erysipelas**: appears similar to cellulitis but the border is distinct and is typically on the face, shin or foot.

### MICRO-facts

**Cellulitis** can appear similar to **deep vein thrombosis**.

## INVESTIGATIONS

- Look for infection source (e.g. broken skin or cracks in-between toes).
- Swab lesions for MC&S.
- Blood cultures.
- Doppler ultrasound to exclude deep vein thrombosis.

### MICRO-facts

**Blood cultures** should be taken with strict aseptic technique to prevent contamination with skin commensals.

## MANAGEMENT

- **Cellulitis**: amoxicillin (oral) and flucloxacillin (oral) or flucloxacillin (intravenous) and benzylpenicillin (intravenous).
- **Erysipelas**: flucloxacillin or co-amoxiclav or erythromycin (penicillin allergy).
- **MRSA**: vancomycin or teicoplanin; patients should be barrier-nursed in a side room and gloves and gown should be worn.

## COMPLICATIONS

- Sepsis.
- Necrotizing fasciitis.

# 13.6 NECROTIZING FASCIITIS

## DEFINITION

- Necrotizing fasciitis is a rapidly spreading and potentially fatal infection of the subcutaneous tissue and underlying fat.

## INFECTIVE AGENTS

- **Type 1 or progressive bacterial synergistic gangrene (multiple agents)**:
    - *Staphylococcus* spp.;
    - Coliforms;
    - *Bacteroides* (Gram-negative non-sporing anaerobic bacilli);
    - *P. aeruginosa* (immunosuppressed).
- **Type 2**: *S. pyogenes*.

## RISK FACTORS

- **Type 1**:
    - abdominal surgery;
    - diabetes mellitus;
    - chronic ulcers.
- **Type 2**: often spontaneous.

> **MICRO-facts**
>
> Consider **necrotizing fasciitis** in all patients with **cellulitis**, especially those who appear very unwell.

## PATHOPHYSIOLOGY

- Infection causes thrombosis in the arterioles that supply the skin.
- Consequently, the skin and fatty tissue becomes ischaemic and later necrotic.
- This process is very rapid and spreads along the tissue planes.

## CLINICAL FEATURES

- **Initially**: cellulitis-like rash or normal appearance (infection is deep).
- **Later**:
    - skin becomes erythematous, painful, oedematous and then necrotic with areas of anaesthesia;
    - fever, sepsis and multiorgan failure.

## INVESTIGATIONS

- Swab lesions for MC&S.
- Blood cultures.

### MANAGEMENT

- **Antibiotics**: piperacillin and tazobactam (Tazocin) and clindamycin.
- **Surgery**: surgical debridement.

### COMPLICATIONS

- Sepsis.
- Death.

## 13.7 GAS GANGRENE (CLOSTRIDIAL MYONECROSIS)

### DEFINITION

- Gas gangrene is a potentially fatal infection of deep tissues by *Clostridium* spp.
- The muscle layers are characteristically targeted.

### INFECTIVE AGENTS

- *Clostridium perfringens* (most common).
- Other *Clostridium* spp. (e.g. *Clostridium septicum*, *Clostridium histolyticum* and *Clostridium tertium*).

### RISK FACTORS

- Open deep wounds and exposure to spores in faeces or soil.
- Peripheral vascular disease.
- Enteric surgery.

### PATHOPHYSIOLOGY

- *Clostridium* spp. produce enzymes that enable them to metabolize the saccharides and proteins found in the deep tissue layers.
- This process results in the destruction of muscle and the production of large amounts of gas, causing swollen gas-filled tissue.
- In addition, *C. perfringens* produces α-toxin, which catalyses the destruction of cell membranes resulting in haemolysis and anaemia.

### CLINICAL FEATURES

- Swollen, painful and discoloured tissue with fluid and gas-filled blisters.
- Tissue crepitus suggests underlying gas.
- Haemolytic anaemia and jaundice.
- Sepsis.

### INVESTIGATIONS

- Clinical diagnosis.
- Swab lesions for MC&S.
- **Full blood count**: anaemia.
- Blood cultures.

> **MICRO-facts**
>
> **Do not delay treatment** waiting for investigation results, **gas gangrene** can be **fatal**.

### MANAGEMENT

- **Antibiotics**: benzylpenicillin or teicoplanin (penicillin allergy) and metronidazole.
- **Surgery**: surgical debridement.

### COMPLICATIONS

- Limb amputation following severe muscle destruction.
- Death.

## 13.8 WOUND INFECTION

### DEFINITION

- All wounds have the potential to become infected; however, surgical wounds are particularly susceptible. This is because they are often large wounds and the post-operative hospital stay may expose patients to a range of pathogens.

### INFECTIVE AGENTS

- *S. aureus.*
- Enterococci.
- Coliforms (e.g. *Escherichia coli*, *Klebsiella* spp. and *Proteus* spp.).
- *P. aeruginosa.*
- *C. perfringens.*

### RISK FACTORS

- **Simple wound infection**:
  - poor wound care;
  - exposure to contaminated areas.
- **Surgical wound infection**:
  - indwelling equipment such as drains and catheters;
  - bowel operations;

- large operation wounds;
- poor healthcare professional hygiene.

### CLINICAL FEATURES

- Peri-wound erythema with pain and pus discharge.
- Fever.

### INVESTIGATIONS

- Swab lesions for MC&S.

### MANAGEMENT

- **Antibiotics**: based on results of laboratory investigations.

### COMPLICATIONS

- Poor surgical wound healing.
- Infection of local tissues.
- Sepsis.

## 13.9 SHINGLES (ZOSTER)

### DEFINITION

- Shingles is caused by reactivation of latent varicella zoster virus and causes a painful rash with a dermatomal distribution.

### INFECTIVE AGENTS

- Varicella zoster virus (latent reactivation following varicella (chickenpox)).

### RISK FACTORS

- Elderly.
- Immunocompromised.

### PATHOPHYSIOLOGY

- Following varicella infection (usually as a child), the virus remains latent in the sensory dorsal root and cranial nerve ganglia.
- Reactivation occurs at a much later date and causes symptoms related to a specific dermatome.

### CLINICAL FEATURES

- Red, painful and unilateral vesicular rash following a dermatomal distribution (classically a band lesion around the thorax but also on the face).
- Lesions eventually become pustular and then form crust.

### INVESTIGATIONS

- Clinical diagnosis; further investigation rarely required.
- Swab lesions for tissue culture or polymerase chain reaction detection of viral nucleic acids.

### MANAGEMENT

- **Antiviral**: aciclovir (reduces pain and complications).

### COMPLICATIONS

- **Post-herpetic neuralgia**: persistent dermatomal pain despite resolution of rash.
- **Secondary infection of lesions**: usually Gram-positive bacteria.
- **Disseminated zoster**: immunocompromised patients.
- **Ophthalmic zoster**: infection of the eye can cause uveitis and keratitis.
- **Ramsay–Hunt syndrome (herpes zoster oticus)**: zoster infection of the seventh and eighth cranial nerves causes earache, facial palsy and zoster vesicles around the ear and on the tympanic membrane.
- **Encephalitis**: rare.

## 13.10 SCALDED SKIN SYNDROME

### DEFINITION

- Scalded skin syndrome is an umbrella term for a group of conditions caused by staphylococcal toxin production.

### INFECTIVE AGENTS

- *S. aureus.*

### TYPES

- **Ritter's disease**: neonates.
- **Toxic epidermal necrolysis or Lyell's disease**: older children and adults.

### PATHOPHYSIOLOGY

- *S. aureus* can produce a protease toxin that damages the epidermis and causes the characteristic skin lesions.
- As scalded skin syndrome is toxin mediated, the original infection can be at a distant site such as the throat.

### CLINICAL FEATURES

- Fragile blisters form on the skin that can be easily removed with pressure (Nikolsky's sign).

- The underlying skin is erythematous and resembles scalds.

## INVESTIGATIONS

- Clinical diagnosis.
- Swab lesions for MC&S.

## MANAGEMENT

- **Antibiotic**: flucloxacillin.

## 13.11 COMMON CHILDHOOD RASHES

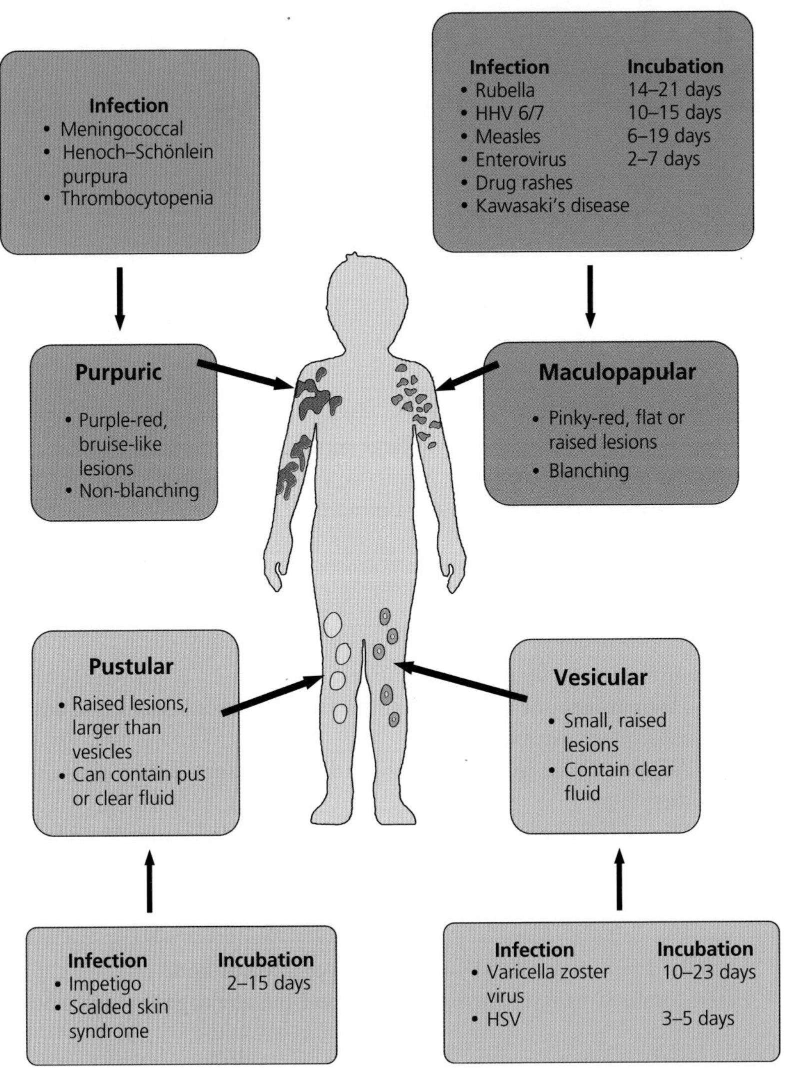


Fig. 13.2 Common childhood rashes. HHV, human herpesvirus; HSV, herpes simplex virus.

# 14 Bone and joint infections

## 14.1 OSTEOMYELITIS

### DEFINITION

- Osteomyelitis is an infection of bone.

### INFECTIVE AGENTS

- Osteomyelitis can be caused by a large number of organisms; the most common pathogens are:
  - *Staphylococcus aureus* (most common);
  - *Streptococcus pyogenes*;
  - coliforms.

### PATHOPHYSIOLOGY

- Infection can occur by three mechanisms:
  - **Haematogenous spread**: distant infection causes bacteraemia and subsequent osteomyelitis.
  - **Adjacent joint infection**: septic arthritis can spread from the joint to the bone.
  - **Direct infection**: trauma, surgery or a deep ulcer can infect adjacent bone.

### CLINICAL FEATURES

- **Initially**: fever, malaise and vague pain over infected bone.
- **Later**: localized pain, erythema, swelling and pus drainage through sinuses.

### INVESTIGATIONS

- Clinical diagnosis.
- Swab pus for microscopy, culture and sensitivity (MC&S).
- Blood culture.
- **Radiograph**: changes only visible after 7–10 days; bone destruction and joint effusions.
- **MRI**: bone destruction, effusions and joint damage.

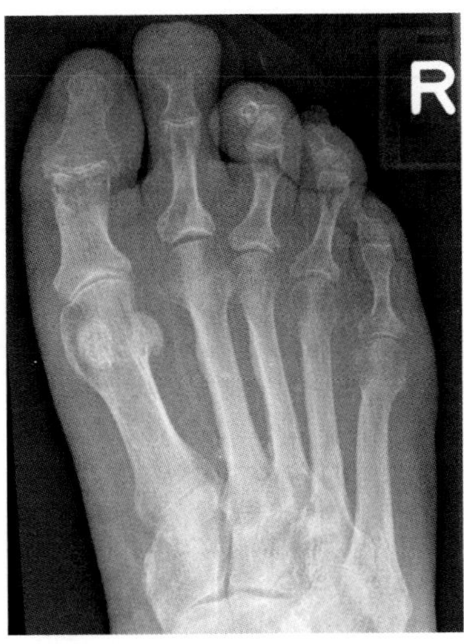


Fig. 14.1 Radiograph of a foot showing destruction of the second distal phalanx due to osteomyelitis. Courtesy of Dr I. Bickle, Northern General Hospital, Sheffield, UK.

### MANAGEMENT

- **General**: immobilize the bone.
- **Medication**: flucloxacillin and fusidic acid (until laboratory results available); long-term treatment required as bony uptake of antibiotics is poor.
- **Surgical**: drainage of pus collections and dead bone (sequestrum).

### COMPLICATIONS

- **Brodie's abscess**: a bony abscess filled with pus but surrounded by sclerotic bone. Increases the risk of future infections.
- **Chronic osteomyelitis**: prolonged infection that causes significant morbidity. Discharging sinuses are commonly found.
- **Prolonged antibiotic therapy**: osteomyelitis demands many weeks of antibiotic therapy and this can predispose patients to other infections such as candidiasis or pseudomembranous colitis.

## 14.2 SEPTIC ARTHRITIS

### DEFINITION

- Septic arthritis is an infection of bone.
- Commonly shoulder, hip and knee.

## INFECTIVE AGENTS

- Septic arthritis can be caused by a large number of organisms; the most common pathogens are:
  - *S. aureus*;
  - *S. pyogenes*;
  - *Haemophilus influenzae* (type b);
  - *Neisseria gonorrhoeae*;
  - *Pseudomonas aeruginosa*;
  - coliforms.

## PATHOPHYSIOLOGY

- Infection can occur by two mechanisms:
  - **Haematogenous spread**: distant infection causes bacteraemia and subsequent septic arthritis.
  - **Direct infection**: trauma, surgery or a deep ulcer can infect an adjacent joint.
- Joint destruction occurs rapidly.

## CLINICAL FEATURES

- Acute onset of a painful, warm, swollen and erythematous joint.
- Patient often isolates the joint to minimize pain.
- **Gonococcal arthritis**: polyarthralgia, tenosynovitis and pustules on distal limbs.

## INVESTIGATIONS

- Aspirate the joint for MC&S.
- **Blood tests**:
  - **Full blood count**: leucocytosis.
  - Blood culture.
- **Imaging**:
  - **Radiograph**: peri-articular soft-tissue swelling.

## MANAGEMENT

- **General**: immobilize the joint and start physiotherapy early.
- **Medication**:
  - **Empirical**: cefuroxime and flucloxacillin (until laboratory results available).
  - **Later**: discuss with microbiologist and switch to appropriate antibiotic.
- **Surgical**: drainage of pus and fluid.

## COMPLICATIONS

- Loss of joint function.
- Death.

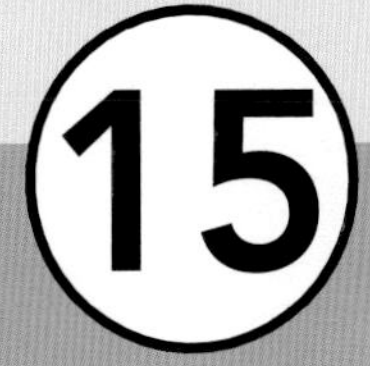

# Congenital, neonatal and childhood infections

## 15.1 CONGENITAL INFECTIONS (TABLE 15.1)

## 15.2 NEONATAL INFECTIONS

### GENERAL INFORMATION

- **Key features**:
  - Infection is commonly transferred from the mother. Accordingly, organisms that can colonize the vagina are the usual culprits.
  - Neonates are unlikely to display classical features of any particular infection so must be watched closely.
- **Infective agents**:
  - **Bacterial**:
    - *Streptococcus agalactiae*;
    - *Listeria monocytogenes*;
    - *Escherichia coli*;
    - *Klebsiella* spp.;
    - *Pseudomonas* spp.;
    - *Staphylococcus aureus*.
  - **Viral**: herpes simplex virus.
- **Diagnosis**: septic screen.
- **Treatment**: dependent upon pathogen.
- **Prevention**: intrapartum penicillin to mothers who are group B *Streptococcus* positive.

### OPHTHALMIA NEONATORUM

- **Key features**: ophthalmia neonatorum is defined as conjunctivitis within the first 28 days of life (neonatal period).
- **Infective agents**:
  - **Bacterial**:
    - *Neisseria gonorrhoeae*;
    - *Chlamydia trachomatis*;
    - *S. aureus*;

Table 15.1 Clinical features of congenital infections

| INFECTIVE AGENT | IMPAIRED HEARING | VISUAL PROBLEMS | COGNITIVE IMPAIRMENT | GROWTH RESTRICTION | PROLONGED JAUNDICE | RASH | HEART DEFECTS | HEPATO-SPLENOMEGALY | INTRACEREBRAL CALCIFICATION | HYDRO-CEPHALUS |
|---|---|---|---|---|---|---|---|---|---|---|
| Rubella | ✓ | ✓ Cataracts | ✓ | ✓ | ✓ | | ✓ | | | |
| Cytome-galovirus | ✓ | | ✓ | ✓ | ✓ | ✓ Petechiae | | ✓ | | ✓ |
| Toxoplasma | | ✓ Chorioretinitis | ✓ | ✓ | | | | | ✓ | ✓ |
| Varicella zoster virus | | ✓ | | | | ✓ Vesicular rash | | | | |
| Syphilis | ✓ | ✓ | ✓ | ✓ | | ✓ Soles and palms | | | | |

  - *Haemophilus influenzae*;
  - *Streptococcus pneumoniae*.
- **Clinical features**:
  - purulent discharge from the eyes;
  - eyelid swelling.
- **Diagnosis**: swab discharge.
- **Treatment**:
  - ***N. gonorrhoeae***: ceftriaxone.
  - ***C. trachomatis***: erythromycin.
  - ***S. aureus***: fusidic acid.
  - **Other**: neomycin (eye drops) or chloramphenicol (eye drops).

## 15.3 CHILDHOOD INFECTIONS

### MEASLES (RUBEOLA)

- **Infective agent**: measles virus.
- **Clinical features**:
  - **Prodrome**: fever, cough, conjunctivitis, coryza and irritability.
  - **Koplik's spots**: white spots on inflamed buccal mucosa (often not seen as fade early).
  - **Rash**:
    - starts behind ears, spreads downwards to whole body;
    - initially maculopapular but later becomes blotchy;
    - fades in 7–10 days.
- **Investigations**:
  - Measles virus immunoglobulin (Ig) M antibody detected by enzyme-linked immunosorbent assay (ELISA) of saliva or blood (1–6 weeks after onset of symptoms).
  - Immunofluorescence for measles antigen.
  - Viral culture of buccal or nasopharyngeal swab.
- **Management**:
  - **General**: supportive, and isolate to prevent spread.
  - **Medication**:
    - **Normal immunity**: no specific treatment available.
    - **Immunocompromised**: ribavirin.
    - **Secondary bacterial infection**: appropriate antibiotics.
  - **Prevention**: measles–mumps–rubella (MMR) vaccine.
- **Complications**:
  - **Secondary bacterial infections**:
    - Significant cause of mortality.
    - **Examples**: pneumonia, otitis media and bronchitis.

- **Encephalitis**: may cause significant sequelae such as seizures, deafness or learning difficulties.
- **Subacute sclerosing panencephalitis**:
  - rare side-effect (1 in 1 000 000).
  - develops 7–10 years after measles infection, commonly among children who had a primary infection before the age of 2 years;
  - a progressive loss of neurological function results in spasticity, seizures and eventually death.

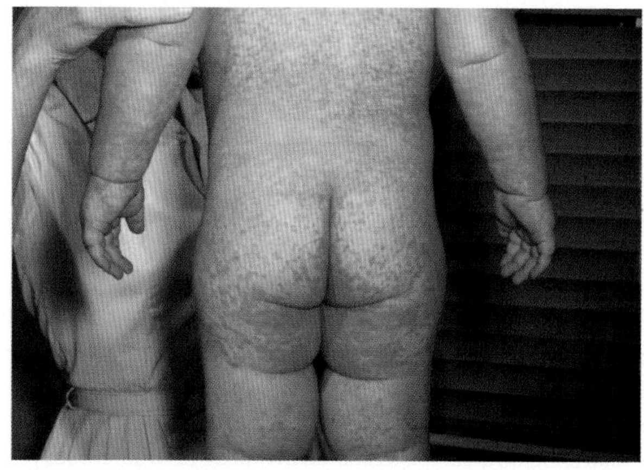

Fig. 15.1 Maculopapular rash of measles infection. Courtesy of the US Centers of Disease Control and Prevention.

## MUMPS

- **Infective agent**: mumps virus.
- **Clinical features**:
  - parotitis (usually bilateral and tender; lasts for 7–10 days);
  - fever.
- **Investigations**:
  - culture of saliva, cerebrospinal fluid or urine sample on monkey kidney cells;
  - polymerase chain reaction (PCR) to detect viral antigen from saliva or urine sample;
  - blood test to detect serum IgM or IgG.
- **Management**:
  - **General**: supportive, bed rest and isolate to prevent spread.
  - **Medication**:
    - no specific treatment available;
    - analgesics.
- **Prevention**: MMR vaccine.

- **Complications**:
  - orchitis (rare in prepubertal patients but can cause infertility);
  - oophritis;
  - meningitis/encephalitis;
  - pancreatitis.

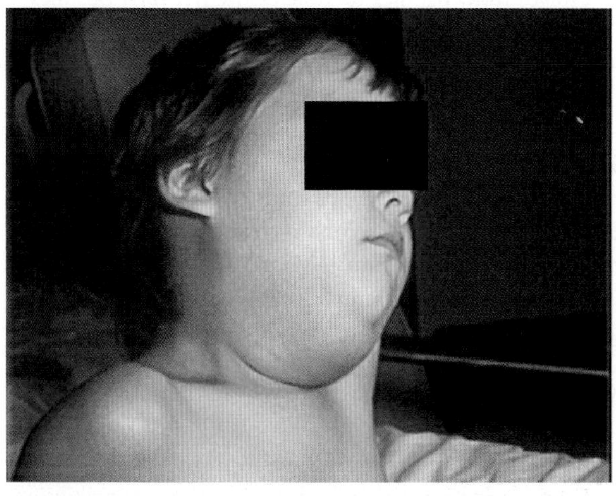

Fig. 15.2 Enlarged parotid glands in mumps infection. Courtesy of the US Centers of Disease Control and Prevention/NIP/Barbara Rice.

## RUBELLA (GERMAN MEASLES)

- **Infective agent**: rubella virus.
- **Clinical features**:
  - **Prodrome**: mild, low-grade fever; malaise; and sore throat.
  - **Rash**:
    - initially erythematous and maculopapular; later becomes confluent;
    - starts on the face and spreads to the whole body;
    - fades in 3–5 days.
  - Lymphadenopathy (suboccipital and post-auricular nodes).
  - Arthralgia.
- **Investigations**:
  - ELISA to detect IgM antibody.
  - PCR to detect viral RNA.
- **Management**:
  - **General**: supportive.
  - **Prevention**: MMR vaccine.

## CHICKENPOX (VARICELLA)

- **Infective agent**: varicella zoster virus.
- **Clinical features**:
  - Fever.
  - **Rash**:
    - evolves from papules to vesicles (itchy); then pustules and finally crusts (eventually fall off, tend not to scar);
    - newer lesions continue to appear so rash will be at different stages;
    - starts on head and trunk and spreads to peripheries.
- **Investigations**:
  - microscopy of vesicles reveals multinucleated giant cells;
  - PCR to detect viral deoxyribonucleic acid;
  - blood test to detect serum IgM or IgG;
  - viral culture of vesicle samples.
- **Management**:
  - **General**: supportive.
  - **Medication**:
    - **Children**: none.
    - **Adolescents/adults/immunocompromised**: aciclovir.
    - **Secondary bacterial infection**: appropriate antibiotics.
  - **Prevention**: varicella vaccine available for non-immune patients at high risk of exposure.

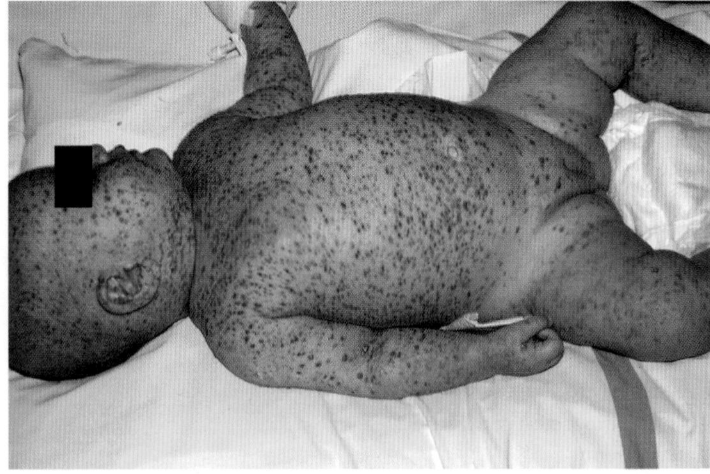

Fig. 15.3 Widespread vesicular chickenpox rash. Courtesy of Dr Hoskyns, Leicester Royal Infirmary, UK.

- **Complications**:
  - secondary bacterial infections;
  - pneumonia;
  - cerebellar ataxia.

## ERYTHEMA INFECTIOSUM (SLAPPED CHEEK OR FIFTH DISEASE)

- **Infective agent**: parvovirus B19.
- **Clinical features**:
  - Fever.
  - **Rash**: erythematous rash on the cheeks (slapped appearance), body and limbs.
- **Management**: supportive as self-limiting.
- **Complications**:
  - **Aplastic crisis**: affects individuals with sickle cell anaemia, hereditary spherocytosis and thalassaemia.

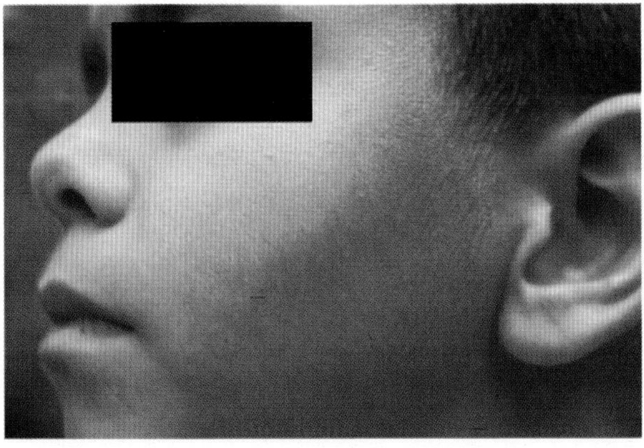

Fig. 15.4 Erythematous rash on the cheeks in erythema infectiosum. Courtesy of the US Centers of Disease Control and Prevention.

## ROSEOLA INFANTUM (EXANTHEM SUBITUM OR SIXTH DISEASE)

- **Infective agent**: human herpesvirus 6 and 7.
- **Clinical features**:
  - Fever and febrile convulsions.
  - **Rash**: generalized macular rash, similar to measles or rubella.
- **Management**: supportive; self-limiting.

## 15.4 UK IMMUNIZATION TIMETABLE

Table 15.2 UK immunization schedule.

| AGE | DISEASES PROTECTED AGAINST | VACCINE |
|---|---|---|
| 2 months | • Diphtheria<br>• Tetanus<br>• Pertussis<br>• Polio<br>• *Haemophilus influenzae* (type b)<br>• *Streptococcus pneumoniae* | • DTaP/IPV/Hib<br>• PCV |
| 3 months | • Diphtheria<br>• Tetanus<br>• Pertussis<br>• Polio<br>• *Haemophilus influenzae* (type b)<br>• *Neisseria meningitidis* (type C) | • DTaP/IPV/Hib<br>• MenC |
| 4 months | • Diphtheria<br>• Tetanus<br>• Pertussis<br>• Polio<br>• *Haemophilus influenzae* (type b)<br>• *Streptococcus pneumoniae*<br>• *Neisseria meningitidis* (type C) | • DTaP/IPV/Hib<br>• PCV<br>• MenC |
| Around 12 months | • *Haemophilus influenzae* (type b)<br>• *Neisseria meningitidis* (type C) | • Hib<br>• MenC |
| Around 13 months | • Measles<br>• Mumps<br>• Rubella<br>• Pneumococcal infection | • MMR<br>• PCV |
| 3 years and four months or soon after | • Diphtheria<br>• Tetanus<br>• Pertussis<br>• Polio<br>• Measles<br>• Mumps<br>• Rubella | • DTaP/IPV<br>• MMR |

Table 15.2 (*continued*)

| AGE | DISEASES PROTECTED AGAINST | VACCINE |
|---|---|---|
| Girls aged 12–13 years | • Human papillomavirus (types 16 and 18) | • HPV |
| 13–18 years | • Tetanus<br>• Diphtheria<br>• Polio | • Td/IPV |

PCV, pneumococcal conjugate vaccine.
Source: http://www.dh.gov.uk/en/Publichealth/Information/index.htm

# 16 History taking, septic screen and monitoring tests

## 16.1 HISTORY TAKING IN INFECTIOUS DISEASES

In addition to the standard medical history, it is also important to enquire about a range of epidemiological risk factors when considering infectious diseases.

- **Travel history**:
  - Has the patient been abroad recently?
  - Where has the patient travelled in the past?
- **Close contacts**: has anyone else in the family or anyone the patient sees regularly been unwell recently?
- **Occupational history**:
  - **Sewage workers**: gastroenteritis, hepatitis and leptospirosis.
  - **Farm workers**: Coxsackievirus and *Coxiella burnetii.*
  - **Abattoir workers**: anthrax.
  - **Sex workers**: genitourinary infections, human immunodeficiency virus (HIV) and hepatitis B.
  - **Health workers**: hepatitis B, respiratory tract infections and gastroenteritis.
- **Hobbies**:
  - **Canoeists**: leptospirosis and gastroenteritis.
  - **Cavers**: histoplasmosis.
  - **Trekkers**: Lyme's disease.
  - **Fresh water swimmers**: schistosomiasis (endemic areas).
  - **Swimming**: cryptosporidia.
- **Pets and animal contact**:
  - **Psittacine birds (parrots)**: *Chlamydophila psittaci.*
  - **Cats**: toxoplasmosis and *Toxocara cati.*
  - **Dogs**: *Toxocara cani.*
  - **Sheep, goats and cattle**: *C. burnetii.*
- **Food and water**:
  - Has the patient eaten any new or different foods recently?
  - Has the patient eaten at a restaurant recently?
  - **Restaurants**: *Salmonella* spp., *Campylobacter* spp. and *Escherichia coli.*

  - **Eggs**: *Salmonella* spp.
  - **Contaminated water**: hepatitis A and E and cholera.
- **Sexual history**: genitourinary infections, HIV and hepatitis B and C.
- **Past medical history**:
  - **HIV**: increased risk of infections (e.g. *Pneumocystis jiroveci* (*Pneumocystis carinii*) pneumonia, toxoplasmosis and candidiasis).
  - **Surgical**:
    - **Splenectomy**: pneumococcal sepsis.
    - **Dentistry**: bacteraemia, increasing risk of endocarditis.
    - **Transplantation**: cytomegalovirus and *Aspergillus* spp.
- **Intravenous drug users**: hepatitis B and C, soft-tissue infections and endocarditis.

## 16.2 SEPTIC SCREEN AND MONITORING TESTS (FIG. 16.1)

## 16.3 STANDARD SEPTIC SCREEN

A standard septic screen includes the following investigations:

- **Observations**: pulse, blood pressure, respiratory rate, temperature and oxygen saturations.
- **Urine sample**: microscopy, culture and sensitivity (MC&S).
- **Stool sample**: culture.
- **Bloods**: culture and full blood count.
- **Imaging**: chest radiograph.
- **Skin/lines**: MC&S ± blood culture of central venous/arterial lines.

## 16.4 MONITORING DURING SEPSIS

### CARDIAC

- **Electrocardiogram**: in this situation, an electrocardiogram has two main roles. First, as a means of distinguishing a tachycardia associated with sepsis from other causes. Second, for diagnosing an atrial fibrillation associated with sepsis.
- **Echocardiogram**: an echocardiogram (transoesophageal is the gold standard) can be used to diagnose endocarditis.

### GASTROINTESTINAL

- **Microscopy**: looking for ova, cysts and parasites.
- **Polymerase chain reaction**: to detect presence of norovirus and *Clostridium difficile* toxin.

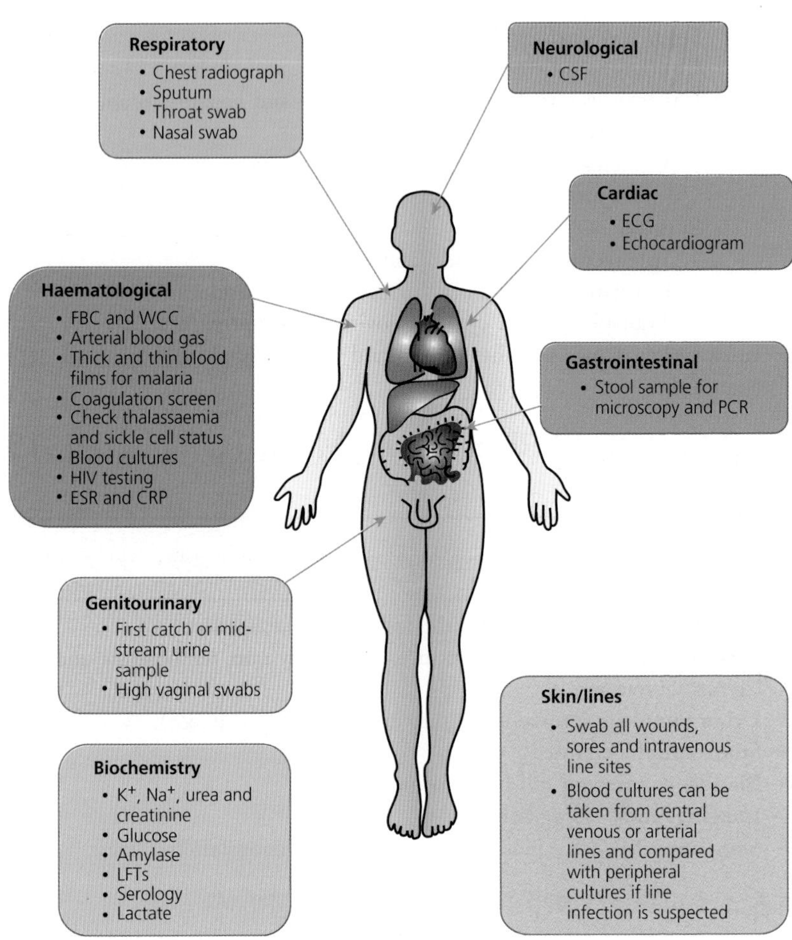


Fig. 16.1 Septic screen and monitoring tests. CRP, C-reactive protein; CSF, cerebrospinal fluid; ECG, electrocardiogram; ESR, erythrocyte sedimentation rate; FBC, full blood count; HIV, human immunodeficiency virus; LFT, liver function test; PCR, polymerase chain reaction; WCC, white cell count.

## HAEMATOLOGICAL

- **Arterial blood gas**: can reveal whether the patient is acidotic owing to high lactate levels associated with sepsis.
- **Erythrocyte sedimentation rate (ESR) and C-reactive protein (CRP)**: both are used to monitor the severity of infection and response to treatment. If these indicators (in combination with the white cell count (WCC)) are not falling after 48 hours of antibiotics, the choice of anti-microbial or presumed source of infection should be reviewed. If CRP, ESR and WCC remain

persistently high after several days of medication, further investigations should be used to rule out endocarditis or a collection (such as a psoas abscess), which may need draining.

## GENITOURINARY

- **Urine samples**: first-catch samples are more useful for genitourinary infections (e.g. chlamydia) whereas mid-stream urine samples are better for urinary tract infection.

## BIOCHEMISTRY

- **Potassium and sodium**: imbalances in relation to infection are commonly from sweating during rigors or diarrhoea and vomiting due to sepsis.
- **Urea and creatinine**: septic shock can cause acute renal failure; therefore, urea and creatinine are useful to monitor renal function. Additionally, urea is a useful prognostic indicator for pneumonia as part of the CURB-65 score (see Chapter 7, Respiratory infections).
- **Glucose**: should be monitored during severe infection, especially in diabetics whose glycaemic control is often erratic during sepsis.
- **Lactate**: an important marker of sepsis severity.
- **Amylase**: may be raised in an infective pancreatitis.
- **Liver function tests**: deranged in infective hepatitis.

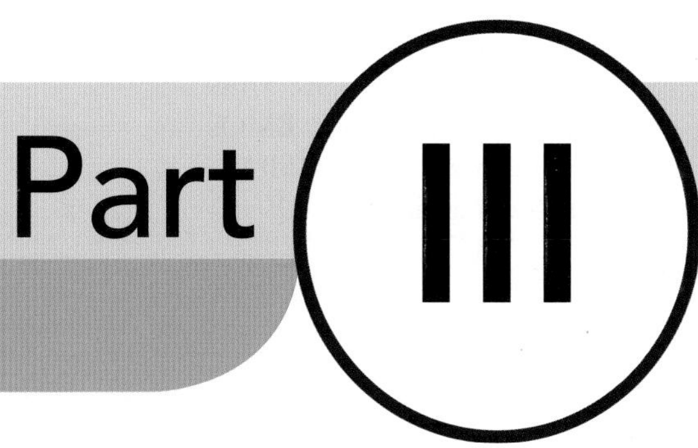


# Self-assessment

# 17 Microbiology

# Questions

## BACTERIA: EMQs

**For each of the following questions, please choose the single most likely bacterium responsible for the presenting conditions. Each option may be used once, more than once or not at all.**

### Diagnostic options

1) *Chlamydia trachomatis*
2) *Neisseria gonorrhoeae*
3) *Neisseria meningitidis*
4) *Staphylococcus aureus*
5) *Staphylococcus epidermidis*
6) *Staphylococcus saprophyticus*
7) *Streptococcus agalactiae*
8) *Streptococcus pneumoniae*
9) *Streptococcus pyogenes*
10) *Viridans* group streptococci

### Question 1

A 7-year-old girl presents to the Accident and Emergency Department with facial swelling, worse around the eyes. A urine sample on admission appears dark and frothy. The patient was treated with oral antibiotics from her GP for a sore throat 2 weeks prior to the onset of the current illness.

### Question 2

A 72-year-old woman is admitted to an infectious diseases ward with headache, photophobia and neck stiffness. Lumbar puncture shows a white cell count of 1000/L, 99% of which were neutrophils, a cerebrospinal fluid (CSF) glucose of 2.1 mmol/L (blood glucose 6 mmol/L) and a markedly elevated protein level. Gram stain shows blue/purple-staining diplococci in the CSF.

### Question 3

A 34-year-old intravenous drug user is admitted with a 2 month history of fevers and rigors. He also has a diastolic murmur, which is found to be tricuspid regurgitation on echocardiography. He had a cardiovascular examination with no abnormal findings 6 months prior to this episode.

**For each of the following questions, please choose the single most likely bacterium responsible for the presenting conditions. Each option may be used once, more than once or not at all.**

## Diagnostic options

1) *Campylobacter jejuni*
2) *Clostridium difficile*
3) *Escherichia coli*
4) *Haemophilus influenzae*
5) *Helicobacter pylori*
6) *Neisseria meningitidis*
7) *Neisseria gonorrhoeae*
8) *Proteus mirabilis*
9) *Shigella dysenteriae*
10) *Vibrio cholerae*

### Question 4

An 85-year-old woman attends her GP surgery with dysuria and increased frequency of micturition. Microscopy of her urine shows a Gram-negative bacillus, which grows in pink colonies on MacConkey agar.

### Question 5

A 53-year-old man presents to a general surgical clinic with epigastric pain. An oesophagogastroduodenoscopy demonstrates a duodenal ulcer, and a *Campylobacter*-like organism (CLO) test, performed at the time, returns a positive result.

### Question 6

A 22-year-old male student presents to the Accident and Emergency Department with severe dehydration, having suffered with vomiting and bloody diarrhoea all day. Two nights prior to admission, he ate with a group of friends in a restaurant with a dubious reputation for hygiene. Another friend has also been unwell, with both patients having eaten a chicken jalfrezi.

**For each of the following questions, please choose the single most likely bacterium responsible for the presenting conditions. Each option may be used once, more than once or not at all.**

## Diagnostic options

1) *Borrelia burgdorferi*
2) *Coxiella burnetii*
3) *Chlamydophila pneumoniae*
4) *Chlamydophila psittaci*
5) *Legionella pneumophila*
6) *Leptospira interrogans*
7) *Mycobacterium leprae*
8) *Mycobacterium tuberculosis*
9) *Mycoplasma pneumoniae*
10) *Rickettsia rickettsii*

### Question 7

A 41-year-old man who has lived in Sheffield, UK, for his whole life presents to his GP with a gradually worsening cough, shortness of breath, fever and malaise.

A chest radiograph shows no focal consolidation, but generalized increased interstitial markings are present, in keeping with atypical pneumonia. On otoscopy the patient's tympanic membranes are erythematous.

### Question 8

A 52-year-old man of no fixed abode is admitted to the Accident and Emergency Department with a cough and shortness of breath. He mentions that he has been unwell for around 6 months, and his cough has gradually worsened over that period. He has also lost more than 1 stone ($\sim$6.25 kg) in weight, and wakes up regularly drenched in sweat. A chest radiograph on admission shows an opacity in the upper lobe of the left lung, and a pleural effusion on that side.

### Question 9

A 35-year-old man is admitted with fever, malaise and hepatomegaly. He also has conjunctival suffusion. He works for the town council as a parks attendant and has spent the summer on a project to clean up local rivers and streams. He frequently wades in sandals, as he finds waders too hot in the English summer weather.

**For each of the following questions, please choose the single most likely bacterium responsible for the presenting conditions. Each option may be used once, more than once or not at all.**

## Diagnostic options

1) *Chlamydia trachomatis*
2) *Haemophilus influenzae*
3) *Klebsiella pneumoniae*
4) *Neisseria meningitidis*
5) *Staphylococcus aureus*
6) *Staphylococcus epidermidis*
7) *Streptococcus agalactiae*
8) *Streptococcus pneumoniae*
9) *Streptococcus pyogenes*
10) *Viridans* group streptococci

### Question 10

A 68-year-old man is admitted to the Accident and Emergency Department with worsening shortness of breath and cough productive of green sputum with a pyrexia of 38.4°C. This is his third admission in the last 3 months and he mentions he usually requires hospital treatment five or six times each winter. He has home oxygen and nebulizers. You take a sputum sample for microscopy and find a Gram-negative coccobacillus.

### Question 11

A 35-year-old man, who has a history of splenectomy for immune thrombocytopenic purpura 2 years ago, presents to the Accident and Emergency Department having collapsed. On examination, he is febrile, with a temperature of 39°C, and is hypotensive. You treat him for septic shock and take samples for blood culture. He admits to being poorly compliant with his medication, and has not attended all of his follow-up appointments.

### Question 12

A 5-year-old boy presents to the GP with a crusty lesion on his face. It is painful, and the patient has been generally unwell with a fever for the last 2 days. The lesion is golden in colour, and the patient's mother explains that several children from the local playgroup have had a similar illness recently.

## BACTERIA: SBAs

**For the following questions, please choose the single best answer from the options given**

### Question 13

A 35-year-old man presents with an insect bite on his right leg that occurred 2 days ago while he was on a holiday in France. The surrounding skin is erythematous, hot and swollen and his temperature is 38.5°C. He feels generally unwell and had a rigor this morning. You take blood cultures and swabs of the lesion and then decide to start antibiotic therapy. Which of the following is the single most appropriate choice of empirical antibiotics?

1) Intravenous benzylpenicillin and flucloxacillin.
2) Intravenous benzylpenicillin and vancomycin.
3) Intravenous co-amoxiclav.
4) Oral amoxicillin and flucloxacillin.
5) Oral co-amoxiclav.

### Question 14

An 83-year-old woman, recovering in hospital after a repair of a fractured neck of femur, develops profuse diarrhoea. She has recently completed a 7 day empirical course of cefalexin for a urinary tract infection. Which of these bacteria is the single most likely cause of her diarrhoea?

1) *Bacillus cereus.*
2) *Campylobacter jejuni.*
3) *Clostridium difficile.*
4) *Clostridium perfringens.*
5) *Escherichia coli.*

# VIRUSES: EMQs

**For each of the following questions, please choose the single most likely virus responsible for the presenting conditions. Each option may be used once, more than once or not at all.**

## Diagnostic options

1) Adenovirus
2) Coronavirus
3) Echovirus
4) Herpes simplex virus type 1
5) Influenza virus
6) Parainfluenza virus
7) Respiratory syncytial virus
8) Rhinovirus
9) Rotavirus
10) Varicella zoster virus

### Question 15

A 35-year-old mother of two presents to the Accident and Emergency Department with neck stiffness and photophobia. She is found to have lymphocytic cerebrospinal fluid on lumbar puncture. For the last 3 days she has been off work looking after her children. They have both missed school because of gastroenteritis, which the GP had said was probably viral in origin.

### Question 16

A 56-year-old man presents to hospital with facial asymmetry. On examination, he has drooping of the right side of his mouth and loss of forehead folds on the same side. He also complains of hearing loss on the right side, and is found to have an erythematous, pustular eruption in his ear canal on otoscopy.

### Question 17

A 70-year-old woman is admitted to hospital with suspected severe community-acquired pneumonia. She is started on treatment with a neuraminidase inhibitor following the result of viral swabs taken on admission.

**For each of the following questions, please choose the single most likely virus responsible for the presenting conditions. Each option may be used once, more than once or not at all.**

## Diagnostic options

1) Coronavirus
2) Epstein–Barr virus
3) Herpes simplex virus
4) Human herpesvirus 8
5) Human papillomavirus
6) Influenza virus
7) Parainfluenza virus
8) Respiratory syncytial virus
9) Rhinovirus
10) Rotavirus

### Question 18

A 35-year-old man, diagnosed with human immunodeficiency virus infection 3 months ago, presents to clinic with a non-tender, purple-coloured lesion on his back. He explains that he has not been taking his highly active anti-retroviral therapy drugs recently because of their side-effects. His CD4 count at diagnosis was 15.

### Question 19

You are a GP and have been asked to review a patient in clinic who presented with tonsillitis to one of your colleagues 3 days ago. The presence of exudate and pyrexia of 38.5°C led the GP to prescribe a 5 day course of oral amoxicillin for the patient. Unfortunately, the man has now developed an itchy maculopapular rash all over his body.

### Question 20

You are working as a junior doctor in the Paediatric Department and are called to see a small child in the Accident and Emergency Department with breathing difficulties. You hear a 'barking' cough from the end of the ward, and find the patient to have stridor on examination.

## VIRUSES: SBA

**For the following question, please choose the single best answer from the options given.**

### Question 21

You are asked to see a 45-year-old woman in the Accident and Emergency Department who works as a bank clerk. She has had a generalized headache for a day, which has gradually worsened. She has some neck stiffness, and you note that she is confused and poorly orientated with a Mini-Mental State Examination score of 15/30. She has mild photophobia and a temperature of 38.5°C. Lumbar puncture demonstrates lymphocytic cerebrospinal fluid and a CT head scan shows an abnormality in the left temporal lobe. Which one of the following viruses is the single most likely cause of her symptoms?

1) Coronavirus
2) Echovirus
3) Herpes simplex virus
4) Influenza virus
5) Varicella zoster virus

## FUNGI, PROTOZOA AND HELMINTHS: SBAs

**For the following questions, please choose the single best answer from the options given.**

## Question 22

A 22-year-old asthmatic student has been unwell for some time. She complains of increased wheeze, fever and cough, and has had several courses of antibiotics and steroids. She remains unwell despite these treatments and mentions to you that she works part time as a gardener. Sputum samples come back positive for fungal growth, and you confirm this with a precipitins serological test. Which is the single most likely cause of her symptoms?

1) *Aspergillus fumigatus*
2) *Candida albicans*
3) *Cryptococcus neoformans*
4) Tinea pedis
5) *Pneumocystis jiroveci*

## Question 23

A 23-year-old medical student on his elective rotation is admitted to hospital in India with severe diarrhoea, flatulence and upper abdominal bloating, present over the last few weeks. He has been working in a rural clinic, drinking tap water and eating local food. Microscopy of the sample demonstrates the presence of flagellated protozoa. Which is the most likely cause of his diarrhoea?

1) *Cryptosporidium parvum*
2) *Entamoeba histolytica*
3) *Giardia lamblia*
4) *Toxoplasma gondii*
5) *Trypanosoma cruzi*

## Question 24

A 35-year-old Ugandan woman presents to the urology clinic with painless haematuria. Urine bacterial culture is negative, and flexible cystoscopy and CT of the kidneys, ureter and bladder have failed to demonstrate any other pathology to cause the symptom. You decide to perform further urine testing and this demonstrates the presence of the parasitic ova. From the list, which is the single most likely cause of the haematuria?

1) *Ascaris lumbricoides*
2) *Enterobius vermicularis*
3) *Necator americanus*
4) *Schistosoma haematobium*
5) *Taenia solium*

## ANTIBIOTICS: SBAs

**For the following questions, please choose the single best answer from the options given.**

### Question 25

A 40-year-old man on a business trip to Pakistan develops diarrhoea after eating street food. The local GP starts him on a DNA gyrase inhibitor. Which is the single most likely treatment started?

1) Amoxicillin
2) Cefalexin
3) Ciprofloxacin
4) Erythromycin
5) Metronidazole

### Question 26

A 27-year-old Somalian man presents to infectious diseases clinic complaining of 'bloody urine'. He has recently started on tuberculosis therapy, but missed his appointment for drug counselling. On inspection, his urine is orange. You believe that he is experiencing a side-effect of his medication; which of the following treatment options is the single most likely cause of his symptoms?

1) Ethambutol
2) Isoniazid
3) Pyrazinamide
4) Rifampicin
5) Streptomycin

### Question 27

A 17-year-old man presents to his GP with severe sunburn. The patient normally tans well, but has recently started a new medication for acne. He spent only a short time in the sun and wonders whether this may be a side-effect of his tablets. Which of the following treatment options is the single most likely cause of his symptoms?

1) Clindamycin
2) Doxycycline
3) Erythromycin
4) Metronidazole
5) Teicoplanin

## Question 28

A 16-year-old girl presents with severe pneumonia. She is known to be allergic to penicillin, and is given a drug from a different class to treat her infection. Shortly after administration of the medication, she becomes wheezy, breathless and notices swelling of her lips. She is treated with adrenaline, steroids, nebulizers and anti-histamine. Which of the following treatment options is the single most likely cause of the patient's adverse reaction?

1) Cefuroxime
2) Co-amoxiclav
3) Doxycycline
4) Erythromycin
5) Vancomycin

## Question 29

A baby with neonatal sepsis is started on empirical antibiotics while a septic screen is performed. The doctors on the special care baby unit take regular blood samples to measure the levels of one of the drugs used as they are worried about side-effects, including ototoxicity and nephrotoxicity. Please choose the single most likely antibiotic treatment that is to be monitored.

1) Benzylpenicillin
2) Ceftriaxone
3) Flucloxacillin
4) Gentamicin
5) Vancomycin

## Question 30

A 26-year-old woman presents to her GP with dysuria and haematuria. She has recently discovered she is pregnant. You are keen to treat her urinary tract infection, but are worried about potential side-effects of antibiotics. Which of the antibiotic treatment options from the list would you definitely avoid?

1) Cefalexin
2) Co-amoxiclav
3) Nitrofurantoin
4) Penicillin V
5) Trimethoprim

# Answers

## BACTERIA: EMQs

### Answer 1

9) ***Streptococcus pyogenes***: this is a history of acute post-streptococcal glomerulonephritis. In epidemics, up to 10% of patients with bacterial pharyngitis go on to develop this complication.[1] Group A -haemolytic streptococci (*Streptococcus pyogenes*) are the most common cause of bacterial pharyngitis, although viral infection is far more common overall. See Chapter 1, Bacteria for further information about streptococci.

### Answer 2

8) ***Streptococcus pneumoniae***: this patient has bacterial meningitis. The most common pathogens causing this illness are *Streptococcus pneumoniae*, *Neisseria meningitidis* and *Haemophilus influenzae*.[2] Both of the two probable causes in this question are diplococci, with *S. pneumoniae* being Gram-positive, and *N. meningitidis* being Gram-negative. The Gram stain result is the key differentiator between the two in this case. In addition, bacterial meningitis is more commonly caused by *N. meningitidis* in younger patients, whereas *S. pneumoniae* is the more likely pathogen in the elderly.[2] See Chapter 1, Bacteria for more information about these bacteria.

### Answer 3

4) ***Staphylococcus aureus***: this patient is likely to have tricuspid valve bacterial endocarditis. *Staphylococcus aureus* is the most likely pathogen in this case. Being a skin commensal, it is often associated with endocarditis in those injecting drugs into their veins. The tricuspid valve is the first of the heart valves to receive blood from the venous system, and is therefore classically the first valve to be affected by a *S. aureus* infection. *Viridans* group streptococci are the most common cause of bacterial endocarditis, and may be associated with recent dental manipulation. *Staphylococcus epidermidis* is associated with prosthetic valve endocarditis.

### Answer 4

3) ***Escherichia coli***: this patient has a urinary tract infection (UTI). Common causes of UTIs included in the possible answers are *Escherichia coli* and *Proteus mirabilis*. Both are Gram-negative bacilli, but only *E. coli* is a lactose fermenter, meaning that it will grow in pink colonies on MacConkey agar. *P. mirabilis* would grow in clear colonies on this medium.

## Answer 5

5) ***Helicobacter pylori***: this man has duodenal ulceration, which is strongly linked to infection with *Helicobacter pylori*. The positive *Campylobacter*-like organism (CLO) test is highly suggestive of this infection. Gastric or duodenal ulcers caused by this bacterium may be treated effectively with triple therapy – high-dose proton pump inhibitor (PPI) with two anti-bacterial agents, usually amoxicillin and metronidazole.

## Answer 6

1) ***Campylobacter jejuni***: *Campylobacter jejuni, Escherichia coli, Vibrio cholerae* and *Shigella dysenteriae* can all cause infective gastroenteritis. Cholera and shigellosis are both contracted via faecal–oral spread, which could have been the route of transmission in this case; however, as chicken is mentioned, the most likely organism is *C. jejuni*. One would also expect watery, rather than bloody, stool with *V. cholerae,* which would be extremely profuse – up to 25 litres in a day. Infection with this organism would be highly unusual in this country. *E. coli* is classically found in undercooked beef.

## Answer 7

9) ***Mycoplasma pneumoniae***: there are several causes of atypical pneumonia in the list, including *Chlamydophila psittaci, Coxiella burnetii, Legionella pneumophila* and *Chlamydophila pneumoniae. Mycobacterium tuberculosis* would also be a possibility, given the radiograph findings, but would be unlikely unless there were epidemiological exposure (i.e. more exotic travel than Sheffield!). Only *Mycoplasma pneumoniae* causes erythema in the tympanic membranes in the context of an atypical pneumonia: a rare, but specific, sign. Otoscopy is a simple bedside test available in a GP surgery; performing it in this case allows appropriate management to be started while diagnostic test results are awaited.

## Answer 8

8) ***Mycobacterium tuberculosis***: this man's history is consistent with pulmonary tuberculosis (TB). The weight loss and night sweats are characteristic of this condition, as is the gradually worsening cough. Homeless people are at an increased risk of TB, and may often present late in their illness. Given this history and chest radiograph findings, the patient should be isolated, ideally in a laminar flow room. While being transferred, he should be given a mask to wear to prevent spread of the bacterium. An important differential would be lung cancer, and should be investigated if *Mycobacterium tuberculosis* were not found in the patient.

## Answer 9

6) ***Leptospira interrogans***: this man has leptospirosis, also known as Weil's disease in the most severe cases. The spirochaete *Leptospira interrogans* is spread via rat urine in fresh water and passes into the body through grazes or mucous membranes. Conjunctival suffusion is erythema of the conjunctivae, without the prurulent exudate that is found in conjunctivitis. It is a characteristic finding in leptospirosis.

## Answer 10

2) ***Haemophilus influenzae***: the patient has chronic obstructive pulmonary disease, and the most common pathogens which cause infective exacerbations of this condition are *Streptococcus pneumoniae, Haemophilus influenzae* and *Moraxella catarrhalis*. As the only Gram-negative coccobacillus, *H. influenzae* is the answer in this case. *Klebsiella pneumoniae* is also a Gram-negative bacillus, but usually causes nosocomial pneumonias.

## Answer 11

8) ***Streptococcus pneumoniae***: this man has pneumococcal sepsis. Patients who have had a splenectomy are at an increased risk of certain infections, particularly those caused by *Streptococcus pneumoniae*. This is due to a decreased ability to produce immunoglobulin M antibodies. Patients are usually immunized against this pathogen, and take anti-bacterial prophylaxis at a low dose, usually penicillin V. This man has not been taking his regular medications and may have missed vaccinations. While several of the other alternatives could cause sepsis, *S. pneumoniae* is the most likely in this case.

## Answer 12

5) ***Staphylococcus aureus***: this boy is suffering with facial cellulitis, and the characteristic golden-coloured, crusty appearance makes *Staphylococcus aureus* the most likely causative organism. This infection is commonly known as impetigo and is easily transmissible, particularly between small children. *Streptococcus pyogenes* often causes cellulitis, but would be unlikely to present with these features. Although not listed in the alternatives, herpes simplex virus would be an important differential should the patient have pre-existing facial lesions, e.g. eczema. This would require intravenous aciclovir treatment.

# BACTERIA: SBAs

## Answer 13

1) ***Intravenous benzylpenicillin and flucloxacillin***: this man has bacterial cellulitis. The most common organisms responsible for this infection are

*Staphylococcus aureus* and *Streptococcus pyogenes.* Benzylpenicillin will cover the *S. pyogenes,* while flucloxacillin will cover *S. aureus.* Vancomycin also covers staphylococci, but would not be started as first-line treatment except in the case of suspected meticillin-resistant *S. aureus* infection. Co-amoxiclav would be an appropriate antibiotic should Gram-negative infection be suspected, e.g. after an animal bite. Both oral options would be inappropriate as the patient is systemically unwell, and therefore requires intravenous therapy. Once they are available, sensitivities from blood cultures and a wound swab should guide future management, e.g. stop flucloxacillin if *S. pyogenes* is found to be the causative organism.

### Answer 14

3) ***Clostridium difficile***: *Clostridium difficile* infection is common in hospital patients, and may be spread from person to person if adequate hygiene precautions are not observed. Any patient suspected to have the infection should be barrier nursed in a side room. Many antibiotics predispose to the development of this infection by altering the patient's natural bowel flora. Broad-spectrum antibiotics such as cefalexin and ciprofloxacin are among the most likely to lead to *C. difficile* and thus should be avoided. In this case, cefalexin is an inappropriate empirical choice of antibiotic for urinary tract infection, and, whatever the organism, 3 days of therapy (usually trimethoprim) is adequate for simple infection. Irresponsible and inappropriate prescribing of antibiotics are important and avoidable causes of hospital-acquired infections.

## VIRUSES: EMQs

### Answer 15

3) **Echovirus**: this patient has viral meningitis. Enteroviruses are the most common cause of this condition, followed by herpes simplex virus 2 (HSV-2), varicella zoster virus then HSV-1.[3,4] The *Enterovirus* group includes poliovirus, Coxsackievirus (A and B), echovirus and numbered enteroviruses. This is a classical history of an *Enterovirus* meningitis, with the virus being contracted from children affected by gastroenteritis caused by the same organism. Although rotavirus and adenovirus also cause diarrhoea in children, they are not common causes of viral meningitis. See Chapter 2, Viruses for further information.

## Answer 16

10) **Varicella zoster virus**: this patient has a lower motor neurone facial palsy. Should an upper motor neurone lesion have been responsible, one would expect forehead sparing. Both herpes simplex virus 1 (HSV-1) and varicella zoster virus (VZV) can cause a facial nerve palsy. In the case of HSV-1, Bell's palsy is usually seen, i.e. facial palsy without a rash. This patient has Ramsay–Hunt syndrome, as he has a facial palsy with an accompanying shingles rash. This may present in the mouth or, as in this case, in the ear. Reactivation of hitherto dormant VZV in the geniculate ganglion leads to this syndrome.[5]

## Answer 17

5) **Influenza virus**: during the H1N1 swine flu pandemic, patients were routinely swabbed for influenza A, B and H1 on admission to hospital should they have symptoms of respiratory illness. Often it can be difficult to distinguish clinically between pure bacterial pneumonia and influenza infection, and it is in fact common to have concomitant infection with both pathogens. Oseltamivir is a neuraminidase inhibitor, better known as Tamiflu, which aims to decrease severity and shorten duration of symptoms. Should evidence be found of bacterial infection, antibiotics would also be employed.

## Answer 18

4) **Human herpesvirus 8**: this man has Kaposi's sarcoma, which is strongly linked to infection with human herpesvirus 8. This is an acquired immunodeficiency syndrome-defining illness, as discussed in Chapter 10, Haematological infections and HIV. Given the extremely low CD4 count, the patient is at risk of developing this condition. Although infection with herpes simplex virus is not uncommon in patients with human immunodeficiency virus, one would expect a lesion caused by this virus to appear ulcerated and to be extremely painful. None of the other options would cause a lesion fitting the above description.

## Answer 19

2) **Epstein–Barr virus**: clinical signs are unreliable to differentiate bacterial from viral tonsillitis. Although the presence of an exudate and high fever are more suggestive of bacterial infection, these signs should not be relied on for diagnosis. Tonsillitis is often caused by a virus, of which Epstein–Barr virus (EBV) is one of the commonest pathogens. Amoxicillin can cause a maculopapular rash when given to those with EBV infection, therefore penicillin V or erythromycin should be used in cases of suspected bacterial tonsillitis. Rhinovirus, influenza virus and parainfluenza virus can all cause viral tonsillitis, but do not provoke the same reaction to amoxicillin.

### Answer 20

7) **Parainfluenza virus**: this child has acute laryngotracheobronchitis, better known as croup. The 'barking' cough and stridor are indicative of this diagnosis. Respiratory syncytial virus is a rarer cause of croup. Although not included in this question, acute epiglottitis, caused by *Haemophilus influenzae* type b, should always be considered in patients with stridor. Although far rarer than croup, it is potentially fatal if left untreated. See Chapter 7, Respiratory infections for further information on these conditions.

### Answer 21

3) **Herpes simplex virus**: this woman has herpes simplex virus (HSV) encephalitis. In meningitis, symptoms such as photophobia and neck stiffness are not usually accompanied by confusion unless the infection has spread systemically and caused sepsis and delirium. As such, encephalitis should be considered in any confused patient with meningism. A positive viral polymerase chain reaction for HSV-1 or -2 on cerebrospinal fluid from lumbar puncture is diagnostic for the condition, and aciclovir should be given empirically in cases of high suspicion of encephalitis. A CT head scan can demonstrate focal encephalitis, often in the temporal region. Electro-encephalogram may show characteristic changes associated with HSV encephalitis, as it can alter temporal lobe function.

## FUNGI, PROTOZOA AND HELMINTHS: SBAs

### Answer 22

1) ***Aspergillus fumigatus***: this patient is suffering with allergic aspergillosis. This is an uncommon condition that may affect those with asthma. *Aspergillus fumigatus* is present in soil, dusts and decaying vegetation. A precipitins test uses antibodies to identify antigens by precipitating them out of solution. Respiratory infection with *Candida albicans*, *Pneumocystis jiroveci* and *Cryptococcus* spp. would be highly unlikely unless the patient were immunocompromised. Tinea pedis is also known as athlete's foot.

### Answer 23

3) ***Giardia lamblia***: both *Entamoeba histolytica* and *Giardia lamblia* are common causes of diarrhoea in developing countries and are spread through infected water or food. Giardiasis causes symptoms typical of small intestinal diseases and resulting fat malabsorption. Amoebic disease is typically a bloody diarrhoea (dysentery-like illness). *Cryptosporidium parvum* may also cause gastrointestinal infection, but, of the three, only *Giardia* is flagellated. Toxoplasmosis is usually an infectious mononucleosis-like illness, while *Trypanosoma cruzi* causes Chagas' disease.

## Answer 24

4) ***Schistosoma haematobium***: schistosomiasis is common in sub-Saharan Africa and leads to an estimated 200 000 deaths per year in that region.[6] It is often contracted through swimming in freshwater lakes. None of these other helminths lead to haematuria, as they mainly affect the gastrointestinal system.

# ANTIBIOTICS: SBAs

## Answer 25

3) **Ciprofloxacin**: there is only one DNA gyrase inhibitor in this list and that is the fluoroquinolone ciprofloxacin. It should be remembered that most cases of traveller's diarrhoea simply require supportive therapy with fluids and electrolytes rather than antibiotic therapy.

## Answer 26

4) **Rifampicin**: this anti-tuberculous drug causes secretions, including mucus, tears and urine, to turn a red/orange colour. Side-effects of the other medications are discussed in Chapter 7, Respiratory infections.

## Answer 27

2) **Doxycycline**: oral antibiotics indicated for treatment of acne include macrolides such as erythromycin and clindamycin, and tetracyclines such as doxycycline. Doxycycline can cause photosensitivity in around 20% of patients.

## Answer 28

1) **Cefuroxime**: the patient has a documented penicillin allergy and therefore may also have sensitivity to cephalosporins. This may be the case in up to 10% of patients. Co-amoxiclav contains amoxicillin, and therefore should not be given in penicillin allergy, and the question states that the drug used was from a different class. Although anaphylactic reactions are possible with most antibiotics, given the known cross-sensitivity between cephalosporins and penicillins, cefuroxime is the most likely answer.

## Answer 29

4) **Gentamicin**: this aminoglycoside is very effective for treating severe Gram-negative infections, and also covers some Gram-positive bacteria. It may be given as empirical therapy in severe sepsis, but needs close monitoring as, in high doses, it may cause deafness and renal failure. Vancomycin is the only other drug in the list that is commonly monitored as it can cause renal impairment and, rarely, ototoxicity. It would be unlikely to be used

empirically unless meticillin-resistant *Staphylococcus aureus* infection was suspected, which is not mentioned in the question.

## Answer 30

5) **Trimethoprim**: this antibiotic is an anti-folate drug, and therefore can cause teratogenicity in pregnancy, particularly if used in the first trimester. Safer alternatives include co-amoxiclav and nitrofurantoin, although this should be avoided near term owing to the small risk of neonatal haemolysis. Cefalexin may be given for urinary tract infection (UTI) in pregnancy but is generally not used as first-line treatment. Penicillin V is unlikely to be useful in UTI.

# 18 Infectious diseases

## Questions

### TUBERCULOSIS: SBAs

**For the following questions, please choose the single best answer from the options given.**

#### Question 31

A 33-year-old man from Somalia presents to the Infectious Diseases Department with a 6 month history of weight loss, night sweats and cough. His chest radiograph shows a granuloma in the upper lobe of the left lung, and is highly suggestive of tuberculosis infection. You are keen to start him on empirical anti-tuberculous therapy, but first you want to get a sample of the bacterium for culture and sensitivities to ensure that the patient is on the correct treatments. Three spontaneous sputum samples fail to show any evidence of acid-fast bacilli on auramine phenol stain. What would be the single most appropriate **next** choice of investigation?

1) Bronchoscopy and bronchoalveolar lavage
2) Interferon $\gamma$ assay, e.g. Quantiferon
3) Induced sputum sample
4) Percutaneous biopsy of granuloma seen on chest radiograph
5) Tuberculin skin test (Mantoux test)

#### Question 32

A 40-year-old woman, currently being treated with quadruple therapy for tuberculosis, develops numbness and tingling in her left hand. From the list, which is the single most likely treatment responsible for her symptoms?

1) Capreomycin
2) Ethambutol
3) Isoniazid
4) Pyridoxine
5) Rifampicin

## Question 33

The pharmacist sees a patient with newly diagnosed pulmonary tuberculosis for drug counselling. As part of the consultation, the patient has an eye test. Which drug from the list below is the single most likely treatment to cause optic neuritis?

1) Cycloserine
2) Ethambutol
3) Isoniazid
4) Rifabutin
5) Rifampicin

# GASTROINTESTINAL INFECTIONS: SBAs

**For the following questions, please choose the single best answer from the options given.**

## Question 34

A 21-year-old man is brought to a medical station in a relief zone in Ethiopia with a pyrexia of 39.5°C. He has felt unwell for a few days and has abdominal pain, headache and a dry cough. On examination, you note his pulse to be 40 beats/minute. From the list of alternatives below, please choose the single most likely cause of the patient's symptoms.

1) *Campylobacter jejuni*
2) *Giardia lamblia*
3) *Salmonella enteritidis*
4) *Salmonella typhi*
5) *Vibrio cholerae*

## Question 35

Several members of a wedding party suffer with vomiting 2–3 hours after their buffet supper. They had a selection of different finger foods, none of which included rice. From the options below, which is the single most likely organism responsible for the outbreak?

1) *Bacillus cereus*
2) *Clostridium difficile*
3) *Escherichia coli*
4) *Shigella dysenteriae*
5) *Staphylococcus aureus*

## VIRAL HEPATITIS: SBAs

**For the following questions, please choose the single best answer from the options given.**

### Question 36

A 27-year-old woman presents with deep, painless jaundice. Her alanine transaminase level is markedly raised and she mentions that she began a relationship with a Chinese man 2 months ago who said that he suffered with a similar complaint some years previously. You suspect that the patient may have acute hepatitis B infection. From the table below, please identify the most likely blood results from serological testing, numbered 1–5.

| | Positive or negative | | | | |
|---|---|---|---|---|---|
| **Antibody/antigen** | **1** | **2** | **3** | **4** | **5** |
| Anti-HBc IgM | – | + | – | – | – |
| Anti-HBc IgG | – | – | + | + | + |
| HBeAg | – | + | – | + | – |
| HBeAb | – | – | + | – | + |
| HBsAg | – | + | – | + | + |
| HBsAb | + | – | + | – | – |

Anti-HBc, anti-hepatitis B core antibody; HBeAb, hepatitis B envelope antibody; HBeAg, hepatitis B envelope antigen; HBsAb, hepatitis B surface antibody; HBsAg, hepatitis B surface antigen; IG, immunoglobulin.

### Question 37

A 40-year-old man presents to his GP with abdominal pain and pruritus. On examination, he is tender in the right upper quadrant and is jaundiced. He mentions that he has recently returned from a holiday in Turkey, where he enjoyed the local shellfish. From the list below, please select the single most likely cause of his illness.

1) Epstein–Barr virus
2) Hepatitis A virus
3) Hepatitis B virus
4) Hepatitis C virus
5) Hepatitis D virus

## HAEMATOLOGICAL INFECTIONS: SBAs

**For the following questions, please choose the single best answer from the options given.**

### Question 38

A 26-year-old Nigerian woman is admitted unwell to the Infectious Diseases Department with a high fever of 40°C and rigors. She has recently returned from a trip to visit family in her home country and admits to not taking anti-malarial prophylaxis. Worried, you start her on intravenous quinine and doxycycline, but, as the nurses are preparing the infusion, her consciousness level drops and she starts to fit. Thick and thin blood films show the presence of malarial parasites in the blood. From the list below, which is the single most likely parasite responsible for the patient's illness.

1) *Plasmodium billbrayi*
2) *Plasmodium falciparum*
3) *Plasmodium malariae*
4) *Plasmodium ovale*
5) *Plasmodium vivax*

### Question 39

Which of the below is not an acquired immune deficiency syndrome-defining illness?

1) Cervical cancer
2) Cryptococcal meningitis
3) Herpes simplex virus type 1 encephalitis
4) Non-Hodgkin's lymphoma
5) Oesophageal candidiasis

## GENITOURINARY INFECTIONS: EMQs

**For each of the following questions, please choose the single most likely organism responsible for the presenting conditions. Each option may be used once, more than once or not at all.**

### Diagnostic options

1) *Candida albicans*
2) *Chlamydia trachomatis*
3) Herpes simplex virus
4) Human papillomavirus
5) *Mycoplasma hominis*
6) *Neisseria gonorrhoeae*
7) *Treponema pallidum*
8) *Trichomonas vaginalis*
9) *Staphylococcus aureus*
10) *Streptococcus pyogenes*

### Question 40

A 19-year-old woman presents with vaginal discharge. It is grey-white in colour and the presence of 'clue cells' is noted on microscopy.

### Question 41

A 45-year-old former sailor presents to the cardiology department with symptoms of dyspnoea and ankle swelling. He is found to be in cardiac failure, with a loud early diastolic murmur best heard over the left sternal edge. On further examination, you note that one of his pupils accommodates, but does not react to light.

### Question 42

A 40-year-old woman with type 2 diabetes mellitus presents to her GP with creamy-coloured vaginal discharge. It is extremely itchy. The woman mentions she has not been taking the medications for her diabetes recently because of diarrhoea.

## GENITOURINARY INFECTIONS: SBAs

**For the following questions, please choose the single best answer from the options given.**

### Question 43

A 25-year-old man presents with an exquisitely painful erythematous ulcer on his penis. He has recently had unprotected sex with a new partner, who admits to having had similar lesions on her vulva on several occasions in the past that have appeared and resolved. On several occasions, she has been helped by aciclovir therapy. Which is the single most likely organism responsible for the lesion from the list below?

1) *Chlamydia trachomatis*
2) Herpes simplex virus
3) Human papillomavirus
4) *Treponema pallidum*
5) *Trichomonas vaginalis*

### Question 44

A 24-year-old woman presents with deep dyspareunia and increased vaginal discharge. She has been treated with antibiotics for genitourinary infections in the past and admits to not always using barrier protection during sex. On this occasion, microscopy of a high vaginal swab sample shows Gram-negative diplococci. Which of the below options is the single most likely cause of her symptoms?

1) *Candida albicans*
2) *Chlamydia trachomatis*
3) *Gardnerella vaginalis*
4) *Neisseria gonorrhoeae*
5) *Trichomonas vaginalis*

## PAEDIATRIC INFECTIONS: EMQS

**For each of the following questions, please choose the single most likely organism responsible for the presenting conditions. Each option may be used once, more than once or not at all.**

### Diagnostic options

1) Adenovirus
2) Coxsackievirus
3) Cytomegalovirus
4) *Haemophilus influenzae* type b
5) Parainfluenza virus
6) Parvovirus B19
7) Respiratory syncytial virus
8) Rhinovirus
9) *Streptococcus pyogenes*
10) *Staphylococcus aureus*

### Question 45

Working as an junior doctor in the Paediatric Accident and Emergency Department you see an 8 month old baby, admitted with shortness of breath and cough. On examination the baby has intercostal and subcostal recession and the chest radiograph shows no focal consolidation, although the lungs are hyperinflated. It is January and you have seen three other similar cases the same day. You arrange a nasopharyngeal aspirate to find the responsible pathogen.

### Question 46

A 5-year-old girl attends her GP surgery with a 3 day history of diarrhoea and vomiting. Several of her classmates have suffered with a similar illness.

### Question 47

A 4-year-old boy is admitted to the Paediatric Accident and Emergency Department very unwell with a fever of 38.5°C and a soft stridor. He is drooling and very quiet, and was well as recently as yesterday.

**For each of the following questions, please choose the single most likely organism responsible for the presenting conditions. Each option may be used once, more than once or not at all.**

## Diagnostic options

1) Epstein–Barr virus
2) Measles virus
3) Mumps virus
4) *Neisseria meningitidis*
5) Parvovirus B19
6) *Staphylococcus aureus*
7) *Streptococcus agalactiae*
8) *Streptococcus pneumoniae*
9) *Streptococcus pyogenes*
10) Varicella zoster virus

### Question 48

As the paediatric junior doctor on call, you admit a 6-year-old boy who is generally unwell and complaining of a headache. He is found to be pyrexial with a temperature of 38.9°C, and you see him in a dark room as he cries loudly on looking at the light. Kernig's sign is positive. You leave the room to answer your bleep, but are called back in by the nurse, who explains she can see a non-blanching rash developing on the child's back.

### Question 49

A 7-year-old girl attends her GP surgery with a maculopapular rash on the back of her neck. She has been unwell with coryzal symptoms for the preceding 3 days and you note some small glistening spots inside her mouth.

### Question 50

A 2-year-old baby is admitted having been found to have areas that resemble burns on his skin. The skin is erythematous and there is peeling of the skin on light pressure. There is no suggestion of burning or scalding in the history from the child's parents.

# Answers

## TUBERCULOSIS: SBAs

### Answer 31

3) **Induced sputum sample**: spontaneous sputum samples are often negative for acid-fast bacilli on smear testing, but may be cultured for *Mycobacterium tuberculosis* nonetheless. In order to increase the likelihood of positive culture, it is sensible to get the best possible sample of the organism before starting empirical therapy should the patient's condition be stable enough to postpone immediate treatment. Induced sputum would be the next appropriate investigation, and allows deep sputum samples to be sent for

microscopy, culture and sensitivity (MC&S). Should this also be negative (after three samples), a bronchoscopy and bronchoalveolar lavage would be the next investigation of choice, although, if it were accessible, biopsy of the granuloma during the procedure would provide tissue for histology and culture. Tissue samples are the gold standard for diagnosis, but as it is invasive and expensive to obtain them, other options should be explored first. Interferon $\gamma$ assays and the Mantoux test demonstrate exposure to tuberculosis but do not give a sample for MC&S.

### Answer 32

3) **Isoniazid**: this can lead to vitamin B6 (pyridoxine) deficiency, which can cause peripheral neuropathies. It is usual for patients to be given pyridoxine supplements while on treatment to reduce the likelihood of this complication. None of the other drugs commonly cause peripheral neuropathies, and capreomycin would not be part of standard quadruple therapy.

### Answer 33

2) **Ethambutol**: this is known to cause a variety of visual problems, including loss of acuity, colour blindness and restriction of visual fields. Severe problems such as optic neuritis and blindness may also occur. As such, patients should have a visual assessment prior to commencing this treatment. None of the other drugs listed commonly cause visual side-effects.

## GASTROINTESTINAL INFECTIONS: SBAs

### Answer 34

4) ***Salmonella typhi***: classically, *Salmonella typhi* causes enteric fever, which presents with a high fever, headache, abdominal discomfort and, occasionally, a sparse rash. The symptoms are due to inflammation in Peyer's patches of the gut, and the endotoxaemia that results from the bacteraemia. From the above list, only *S. typhi* causes enteric (typhoid) fever, which presents with a fever and bradycardia, rather than the tachycardia one would expect in sepsis or dehydration.

### Answer 35

5) ***Staphylococcus aureus***: of the bacteria listed, only those that produce either spores or toxins could have caused the outbreak because of the short timescale. *Clostridium difficile* is associated with recent antibiotic use and is therefore unlikely in this case. *Bacillus cereus* is a spore-forming organism, but is typically found in precooked rice which has not been thoroughly reheated. *Staphylococcus aureus* toxin may contaminate food if those preparing the meal have infected skin lesions on their hands. *Escherichia coli*

and *Shigella dysenteriae* are unlikely to cause symptoms within such a short timeframe.

## VIRAL HEPATITIS: SBAs

### Answer 36

2) **Acute hepatitis B infection**: each alternative reflects a different state of hepatitis B infection or immunity. Option 1 is a surface antibody carrier, meaning the patient has been previously immunized against the infection. Option 2 shows acute infection, characterized by the presence of envelope and surface antigens, and the IgM antibody against the core antigen. With time, all patients will develop anti-HBc IgG, which can be used to diagnose previous infection. Option 3 is a patient who has previously had hepatitis B, but is now completely immune and non-infective, having developed antibodies to all three antigens. Options 4 and 5 are carriers with high and low infectivity respectively. The presence of envelope antigen confers a higher rate of infectivity, and, being carriers, both options are HBsAg positive. See Chapter 8, Gastrointestinal infections for more information on this condition.

### Answer 37

2) **Hepatitis A virus**: this man is suffering from acute hepatitis A infection. It is transmitted via the faecal–oral route in contaminated water, with shellfish commonly being the culprit. Although the other four options are all possibilities, a more detailed history would be required to identify risk factors for these conditions. In this case, the history is typical for hepatitis A virus. Vaccination should be offered to those travelling to areas with a high prevalence of the virus.

## HAEMATOLOGICAL INFECTIONS: SBAs

### Answer 38

2) ***Plasmodium falciparum***: this woman could be infected by any of options 2–5, but, given the severity of illness, the most likely parasite is *Plasmodium falciparum*. This is also the commonest parasite in Africa. *Plasmodium billbrayi* does not cause malaria in humans.

### Answer 39

3) **Herpes simplex virus type 1 encephalitis**: a patient with known human immunodeficiency virus (HIV) infection who develops any of the other four options should be considered as having acquired immune deficiency syndrome (AIDS), pending an up-to-date CD4 count. Patients with these

conditions not known to have HIV infection should be offered screening. Aseptic (viral) meningitis or encephalitis is a clinical indicator disease for HIV infection, as listed in the BHIVA guidelines on HIV testing.[7] Although not an AIDS-defining illness, all patients with this condition should still be offered an HIV test.

## GENITOURINARY INFECTIONS: EMQs

### Answer 40

5) ***Mycoplasma hominis***: clue cells are a feature of bacterial vaginosis, which may be caused by *Mycoplasma hominis, Gardnerella vaginalis* or *Bacteroides* spp. See Chapter 5, Genitourinary infections for more information.

### Answer 41

7) ***Treponema pallidum***: this gentleman has signs and symptoms of aortic regurgitation, which may be seen in tertiary syphilis as the infection leads to aortic root dilatation. He has an Argyll Robertson pupil, which is a manifestation of neurosyphilis. The clue is in the occupation: examiners love stereotypes, and, in medical examinations, a sailor is almost invariably infected with syphilis!

### Answer 42

1) ***Candida albicans***: vaginal candidiasis is common in diabetic patients, particularly those with poor control. This woman is most likely taking metformin, which may cause diarrhoea. Although *Candida* infection may be readily treated with anti-fungals such as clotrimazole, improved glycaemic control will also help prevent the condition in diabetic patients.

## GENITOURINARY INFECTIONS: SBAs

### Answer 43

2) **Herpes simplex virus**: this patient has genital herpes. *Chlamydia trachomatis* and *Trichomonas vaginalis* do not cause skin lesions. Human papillomavirus causes genital warts, which do not match the description above. *Treponema pallidum* causes syphilis, which may present with a primary chancre, but this is not overly painful, unlike a herpes lesion which is excruciatingly tender. Mucosal ulceration may occur in secondary syphilis, but this would be unlikely to follow the relapsing and remitting pattern described above. Anti-viral medication such as aciclovir would not help treat syphilis; it would require penicillin therapy.

### Answer 44

4) ***Neisseria gonorrhoeae***: this young woman has symptoms that could indicate infection with most of the above organisms. However, the only Gram-negative diplococcus in the list is *Neisseria gonorrhoeae.*

## PAEDIATRIC INFECTIONS: EMQs

### Answer 45

7) **Respiratory syncytial virus**: this child has bronchiolitis, which is extremely common in the winter months. Respiratory syncytial virus most often causes this, although adenovirus and parainfluenza virus may also precipitate the condition. Treatment is supportive, and diagnosis is made clinically and with the aid of nasopharyngeal aspiration.

### Answer 46

1) **Adenovirus**: this causes several illnesses, including conjunctivitis, bronchiolitis and gastroenteritis. Viral gastroenteritis is far more common than bacterial, and occurs in outbreaks in young children. None of the other options commonly cause the condition.

### Answer 47

4) ***Haemophilus influenzae* type b**: this child has acute epiglottitis, now rare because of the Hib vaccination programme. The key differential here is croup, most commonly caused by parainfluenza virus. Croup has a longer disease course, with coryza preceding more severe symptoms such as stridor. The stridor in croup is harsh and described as 'barking', and you would expect the child to be much more well than this patient. If there is any suspicion of acute epiglottitis, a third-generation cephalosporin such as cefotaxime should be given without delay and senior help should be involved as soon as possible. Whilst *Streptococcus pyogenes* causes tonsillitis/pharyngitis, it is not a cause of acute epiglottitis. See Chapter 7, Respiratory infections for more information.

### Answer 48

4) ***Neisseria meningitidis***: this patient has meningococcal septicaemia. He also has meningitis, almost certainly caused by the same organism. The purpuric rash is characteristic of this condition. See Chapter 12, Nervous system infections for more information on meningitis and meningococcal sepsis.

### Answer 49

2) **Measles virus**: this child has measles, which has a characteristic maculopapular rash and may cause Koplik's spots – white spots on the buccal

mucosa. The infection has been more common since the controversy surrounding the measles–mumps–rubella vaccine.

## Answer 50

6) ***Staphylococcus aureus***: this child has staphylococcal scalded skin syndrome. This may occur in *Staphylococcus aureus* infection and is a result of toxin secreted by the bacteria. The peeling of the skin on gentle pressure is known as Nikolsky's sign.

### MICRO-reference


1. Stetson CA, Rammelkamp CH Jr, Krause RM, *et al.* Epidemic acute nephritis: studies on etiology, natural history, and prevention. *Medicine (Baltimore)* 1955; **34**: 431–50.
2. Gjini AB, Stuart JM, Lawlor DA, *et al.* Changing epidemiology of bacterial meningitis among adults in England and Wales 1991–2002. *Epidemiol Infect* 2006; **134**: 567–9.
3. Kupila L, Vuorinen T, Vainionpää R, *et al.* Etiology of aseptic meningitis and encephalitis in an adult population. *Neurology* 2006; **66**: 75–80.
4. Logan SA, MacMahon E. Viral meningitis. *BMJ* 2008; **336**: 36–40.
5. Sweeney CJ, Gilden DH. Ramsay Hunt syndrome. *J Neurol Neurosurg Psychiatry* 2001; **71**: 149–54.
6. Engels D, Chitsulo L, Montresor A, Savioli L. The global epidemiological situation of schistosomiasis and new approaches to control and research. *Acta Trop* 2002; **82**: 139–46.
7. British HIV Association, British Association of Sexual Health and HIV, British Infection Society. *UK national guidelines for HIV testing 2008.* London, UK: BHIVA, 2008. Available from: http://www.bhiva.org/HIVTesting2008.aspx

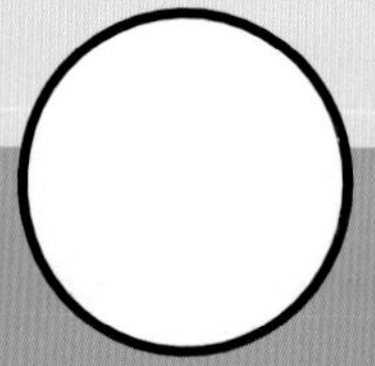

# APPENDIX Notifiable diseases

By law, UK doctors must report cases of the following infections to the Health Protection Agency:

- acute encephalitis;
- acute infectious hepatitis;
- acute meningitis;
- acute poliomyelitis;
- anthrax;
- botulism;
- brucellosis;
- cholera;
- diphtheria;
- enteric fever (typhoid or paratyphoid fever);
- food poisoning;
- haemolytic uraemic syndrome;
- infectious bloody diarrhoea;
- invasive group A streptococcal disease and scarlet fever;
- Legionnaires' disease;
- leprosy;
- malaria;
- measles;
- meningococcal septicaemia;
- mumps;
- plague;
- rabies;
- rubella;
- severe acute respiratory syndrome;
- smallpox;
- tetanus;
- tuberculosis;
- typhus;
- viral haemorrhagic fever;
- whooping cough;
- yellow fever.

# Index

Note: Page numbers with brackets e.g. 211-14(220-3), are to questions with the answer indicated in brackets.

Microbiology

Microbiology

Microbiology